I0812249

Currency Features for Visually Impaired People

Committee on
Currency Features Usable by the Visually Impaired

National Materials Advisory Board
Commission on Engineering and Technical Systems
National Research Council

Publication NMAB-478
National Academy Press
1995

NOTICE: The project that is the subject of this report was approved by the Governing Board of the National Research Council, whose members are drawn from the councils of the National Academy of Sciences, the National Academy of Engineering, and the Institute of Medicine. The members of the committee responsible for the report were chosen for their special competencies and with regard for appropriate balance.

This report has been reviewed by a group other than the authors according to procedures approved by a Report Review Committee consisting of members of the National Academy of Sciences, the National Academy of Engineering, and the Institute of Medicine.

The National Academy of Sciences is a private, nonprofit, self-perpetuating society of distinguished scholars engaged in scientific and engineering research, dedicated to the furtherance of science and technology and to their use for the general welfare. Upon the authority of the charter granted to it by the Congress in 1863, the Academy has a mandate that requires it to advise the federal government on scientific and technical matters. Dr. Bruce Alberts is president of the National Academy of Sciences.

The National Academy of Engineering was established in 1964, under the charter of the National Academy of Sciences, as a parallel organization of outstanding engineers. It is autonomous in its administration and in the selection of its members, sharing with the National Academy of Sciences the responsibility for advising the federal government. The National Academy of Engineering also sponsors engineering programs aimed at meeting national needs, encourages education and research, and recognizes the superior achievements of engineers. Dr. Robert M. White is president of the National Academy of Engineering.

The Institute of Medicine was established in 1970 by the National Academy of Sciences to secure the services of eminent members of appropriate professions in the examination of policy matters pertaining to the health of the public. The Institute acts under the responsibility given to the National Academy of Sciences by its congressional charter to be an adviser to the federal government and, upon its own initiative, to identify issues of medical care, research, and education. Dr. Kenneth I. Shine is President of the Institute of Medicine.

The National Research Council was organized by the National Academy of Sciences in 1916 to associate the broad community of science and technology with the Academy's purposes of furthering knowledge and advising the federal government. Functioning in accordance with general policies determined by the Academy, the Council has become the principal operating agency of both the National Academy of Sciences and the National Academy of Engineering in providing services to the government, the public, and the scientific and engineering communities. The Council is administered jointly by both Academies and the Institute of Medicine. Dr. Bruce Alberts and Dr. Robert M. White are chairman and vice chairman, respectively, of the National Research Council.

The study by the National Materials Advisory Board was conducted under Contract No. TEP-92-58(N) with the U.S. Treasury Department, Bureau of Engraving and Printing.

The complete volume of Currency Features for Visually Impaired People is available for sale from the National Academy Press, 2101 Constitution Avenue, NW. Washington, DC 20418. Braille and large print copies of the report may be obtained from The Lighthouse, Inc., 111 East 59th Street, New York, NY 10022. The report is also accessible on the World Wide Web at http://www.nas.edu/.

Library of Congress Catalog Card Number 94-69234.
International Standard Book Number 0-309-05194-0.

Copyright 1995 by the National Academy of Sciences. All rights reserved.
Printed in the United States of America.

COMMITTEE ON
CURRENCY FEATURES USABLE BY THE VISUALLY IMPAIRED

NORBERT S. BAER, *Chair*, New York University, New York
GARY A. BAUM, James River Corporation, Neenah, Wisconsin; North Carolina State University, Raleigh
JOHN BRABYN, Smith-Kettlewell Eye Research Institute, San Francisco, California
JOSEPH GAYNOR, Innovative Technology Associates, Ventura, California
JOHN HASLOP, Thomas De La Rue, Ltd., Hampshire, England
GORDON E. LEGGE, University of Minnesota, Minneapolis
ROBERT R. SHANNON, University of Arizona, Tucson
GLENN T. SINCERBOX, IBM Research Division, Almaden Research Center, San Jose, California

Liaison Representative

SARA CHURCH, Department of the Treasury, Bureau of Engraving and Printing, Washington, D.C.

National Materials Advisory Board Staff

SANDRA HYLAND, Staff Officer
JANICE M. PRISCO, Senior Project Assistant

ACKNOWLEDGMENTS

The Committee on Currency Features Usable by the Visually Impaired would like to acknowledge the contributions of the individuals who made presentations or submitted statements at the workshop held in March, 1994. The information presented helped the committee to understand the needs of the various communities of people who are blind and those with low vision. The understanding that the committee gained about the state of research in visual and tactile perception assisted them in judging proposed currency features against firm technical criteria.

The committee acknowledges the following persons representing groups of blind and visually disabled people for their input in their areas of specialization:

Mr. George Abbott, Randolph-Sheppard Foundation: needs of the blind vendor community

Mr. Dominick D. Bax, The Jewish Guild for the Blind: needs of blind and visually disabled individuals, especially in rehabilitation programs

Ms. Cherie Hendricks: currency identification system

Ms. Billie Jean Hill, American Council of Citizens with Low Vision: needs of the low- vision communities

Mr. Stephen King, Royal National Institute for the Blind: approaches used by the United Kingdom and the European Union

Mr. Marc Maurer, National Federation of the Blind: needs of the blind community

Mr. Oral Miller, American Council of the Blind: needs of the blind community

Ms. Kathleen Monroe, Retinitis Pigmentosa Foundation (RP): changes in vision with RP progression, needs of the RP community

Mr. J. F. Oschwald: currency identification system

Mr. Brian Wallach, The Lighthouse, Inc.: needs of the blind community

The committee acknowledges the following representatives of the research community:

Dr. Aries Arditi, Lighthouse Research Institute: color contrast for target identification

Professor Ian Bailey, University of California, Berkeley: visual target identification

Professor Karlene Ball, Western Kentucky University: vision changes with aging, design for visual target perception

Professor Roger Cholewiak, Princeton University: vibrotactile perception
Professor James Craig, Indiana University: tactile perception
Professor Emerson Foulke, Braille Research Center and University of Louisville: readability of braille and tactile symbols
Dr. Sam Genensky, Center for the Partially Sighted: low-vision population statistics
Professor Morton Heller, Winston-Salem University: tactile perception
Professor Gary Rubin, Lions Vision Center, Johns Hopkins University: vision changes with aging
Dr. Elliot Schreier, American Foundation for the Blind: low-vision population statistics, devices for currency identification

The committee would like to acknowledge the generosity of the following representatives of foreign banks and currency printing authorities in sharing information on their methods and experiences in manufacturing banknotes with various features that can be used by visually disabled people:

Mr. W. Farber, Security Printing Works, Oesterreichische Nationalbank, Austria
Mr. H. Blanckaert and Mr. J. Renders, Département Imprimerie, Banque National de Belgique, Belgium
Mr. Donald Bennett, Department of Banking Operations, Bank of Canada
Ms. Micheline Lefebvre-Manthorp, Bank of Canada
Mr. Rafael Cruz V., Subgerente Industrial, Banco de la República, Colombia
Mr. Alex Jarvis, Bank of England Printing Works
Mr. J. Faou, Service de l'Imprimerie, France
Mr. Sándor Péterfi, Hungarian Banknote Printing Corporation
Mr. E. Soekarna, Indonesian Government Security Printing and Minting Company
Mr. Shlomo Sirkis, Currency Department, Bank of Israel
Mr. Yoshio Minoshima, General Coordination Division, Printing Bureau, Japan
Ing. Luis. J. Marentes M., Banco de Mexico
Mr. A. Benali and **Mr. M. Iraqi**, Bank Al-Maghrib, Morocco
Dr. Peter Koeze, De Nederlandsche Bank, The Netherlands
Mr. Jan Erik Johansen and Mr. Johs. Bjørgo, Norges Bank Seddeltrykkeri, Norway
Mr. Jaime Gaiteiro, Fabrica National de Moneda y Timbre, Spain
Mr. Tommy Blomberg, Printing Division, AB Tumba Bruk, Sweden
Mr. P. Trachsel and Mr. M. Meroni, Banque Nationale Suisse, Switzerland
Mr. Oscar Knapp, Embassy of Switzerland
Mr. Chumpol Santipong, Bank of Thailand
The Director and Assistant Director of the Branch of the Banknote Printing Plant, Central Bank of Turkey

Special recognition goes to Smith-Kettlewell Eye Research Institute, San Francisco, and its staff, for hosting a meeting and tour of their research facility for the committee.

The following members of the Minnesota Laboratory for Low Vision Research are acknowledged for their contributions to measurements conducted by a member of the committee:

Dr. J. Stephen Mansfield, Mr. Andrew Luebker, and Ms. Kaya Garcia. Thanks also go to the following employees of the James River Corporation who participated in a brainstorming session on features: Mr. Robert Aloisi, Mr. Robert Patterson, Mr. Daniel Geddes, and Mr. Donald Voas. The committee also wishes to thank Mr. Steve McGregor of Thomas De La Rue, Inc., for his painstaking compilation of the data contained in Appendix D.

The Lighthouse, Inc. kindly agreed to make this report available to braille readers by printing the entire text of the report in braille format. The Lighthouse will also provide copies of the report in large print on request. We thank The Lighthouse, Inc., and also Mr. Brian Wallach, who was responsible for arranging the special Lighthouse printing.

The committee is particularly grateful to the Bureau of Engraving and Printing's liaison representative, Dr. Sara Church, Office of Advanced Counterfeit Deterrence, for her active participation at all data-gathering meetings and for providing valuable supporting materials and data for the committee's use.

The committee gratefully acknowledges the vital support and contributions of Dr. Sandra Hyland, staff officer at the National Materials Advisory Board, throughout the study; Dr. Robert Schafrik, director of the National Materials Advisory Board, who provided insight and help during the preparation of the report. The committee also thanks Ms. Janice Prisco, who provided much appreciated assistance and administrative support.

PREFACE

Since October 1, 1877, the Bureau of Engraving and Printing (BEP) of the Department of Treasury has printed all U.S. banknotes. The current design of U.S. banknotes has not changed significantly since 1929. In 1990 the New Currency Design Task Force was formed by the Advanced Counterfeit Deterrence Steering Committee, an interagency group including representatives from the Department of the Treasury, the Federal Reserve, the BEP, and the Secret Service. This task force was charged with redesigning the banknotes to make them more difficult to counterfeit. The designs were to be presented to the Secretary of the Treasury for consideration. Initial concepts were announced by the BEP and the Department of Treasury in conjunction with hearings by the U.S. House of Representatives Committee on Banking, Finance, and Urban Affairs on July 13, 1994 (BEP, 1994).

In 1992, the Department of the Treasury requested that the National Research Council, through its National Materials Advisory Board, analyze and recommend counterfeit-deterrence features that could be incorporated into a redesign of U.S. banknotes. Previous studies by the board had assessed counterfeit-deterrence features at times when a major redesign was not anticipated (NRC, 1985, 1987). The study whose major conclusions are summarized in Appendix B (NRC, 1993) focused on the identification of security features that could be used to deter counterfeiting by "casual" and "professional" counterfeiters making use of the enhanced capabilities of the new generation of color copiers and digital copiers and printers.

The BEP recognized that the occasion of a redesign of the U.S. banknotes presented an opportunity to reexamine the issue of making the banknotes more readily usable by people who are visually disabled, an issue it had studied previously (BEP, 1983) at a time when no general redesign was anticipated. The BEP requested that the National Materials Advisory Board extend its study of currency features to features that could assist visually disabled people to more easily handle paper money in a variety of cash transactions. The objectives of the current study were to:

- assess features that could be used by people who are visually disabled to recognize, denominate, and authenticate banknotes;
- recommend features that could be reasonably incorporated into U.S. banknotes using available technology;
- suggest strategies that should be instituted to make the recommended features most effective; and

• identify research needs in particularly promising areas that could lead to attractive future approaches.

Eight volunteers with expertise in advanced reprographic technology, materials science, substrate materials, currency production, psychophysics, optical engineering, chemical engineering, optics, and physics formed the Committee on Currency Features Usable by the Visually Impaired. Two members of the committee conduct research on topics related to visual disabilities and with visually disabled people; one member of the committee is visually impaired. The committee met four times between February and August 1994.

Invited presentations from experts in visual and tactile perception and from representatives of organizations of blind people and people who are visually impaired provided relevant data at a workshop. Information specific to the manufacture and usefulness of various features usable by visually disabled people for denominating banknotes was solicited from representatives of thirty-eight issuing authorities. Eighteen of these representatives responded with information on their experiences producing and using such features as size-denominated banknotes, color, large numerals, and tactile markings. Where appropriate, the information provided by these representatives is cited and is listed in the references as a "personal communication" to the committee.

The committee recognized that reliable denomination of banknotes is essential to maintaining independence for visually disabled individuals. Authentication of banknotes will certainly require features in addition to those added to the banknote for aiding denomination by visually disabled people.

In this report, the committee reviews and assesses possible banknote features for blind and visually disabled people. The scope of the task was limited to consideration of the use of U.S. paper money only, and the committee did not offer an evaluation of the entire circulating medium. Conclusions and recommendations are presented to assist the BEP and the U.S. Treasury Department in developing the design of the next-generation banknotes to ensure that U.S. banknotes are made conveniently usable by the broadest cross-section of the nation's population under a wide range of use conditions. Because of the confidential nature of banknote design and manufacture, the committee was unable to fully assess the costs of, and difficulties associated with, implementation of any of the features recommended and, thus, does not offer a full cost–benefit analysis or a detailed implementation strategy for any features. Due to the fact that some readers may not be familiar with many of the technical terms used, a glossary is provided at the end of the report for their convenience.

In considering the needs of the 3.7 million U.S. citizens with low vision, the committee observed that many documents issued by government agencies, such as passports, stamps, tax forms, and food stamps, could better serve those with low vision if features similar to those discussed in the report were incorporated in their design. Indeed, in some cases, features not considered sufficiently robust for application in banknote design might find early application in other government documents. Similarly, the public education campaign accompanying any introduction of banknote features for visually disabled people should encourage the private sector to include such considerations in packaging design and related applications.

The Executive Summary is reproduced in Appendix A in larger type (15-point) in accordance with guidelines set by the U.S. Postal Service to categorize reading material for legally blind people. A braille or a large-print version of the entire report may be obtained from the Lighthouse, Inc., which can be contacted at (212) 821-9200. Because the braille version of this report will not contain the figure graphics, the figure contents are described in detail in the text. This report may also be accessed via the National Academy of Sciences World Wide Web server at http://www.nas.edu/.

Any comments or suggestions that readers wish to make about the report can be sent via Internet electronic mail to nmab@nas.edu or by fax to the National Materials Advisory Board at (202) 334-3718. Comments on the new banknote design may be addressed by calling the Office of Communications, Bureau of Engraving and Printing, at (202) 874-3019.

Norbert S. Baer, Chair
Committee on Currency Features Usable by the Visually Impaired

REFERENCES

BEP (Bureau of Engraving and Printing). 1983. A Study of Mechanisms for the Denomination of U.S. Currency by the Blind or Visually Impaired. Bureau of Engraving and Printing report to Congressman Edward R. Roybal, Chairman of the U.S. House of Representatives Select Committee on Aging.

BEP (Bureau of Engraving and Printing). 1994. Bureau of Engraving and Printing presentation to the U.S. House of Representatives Committee on Banking, Finance and Urban Affairs, July 13, 1994.

NRC (National Research Council). 1985. Advanced Reprographic Systems: Counterfeiting Threat and Deterrent Measures. National Materials Advisory Board, NRC. Washington, D.C.: National Academy Press.

NRC (National Research Council). 1987. Counterfeit Threats and Deterrent Measures. National Materials Advisory Board, NRC. Washington, D.C.: National Academy Press.

NRC (National Research Council). 1993. Counterfeit Deterrent Features for the Next-Generation Currency Design. National Materials Advisory Board, NRC. Washington, D.C.: National Academy Press.

CONTENTS

LIST OF ILLUSTRATIONS

TABLES

FIGURES

Currency Features

for

Visually Impaired People

EXECUTIVE SUMMARY

There are an estimated 3.7 million people in the United States who are visually disabled, that is, who have corrected visual acuity no better than 20/70[1] in the better eye or who have a maximum visual field of no more than 30 degrees (Genensky, 1994). About 200,000 of these people are blind (have no useful pattern vision), and 3.5 million have low vision. The leading causes of low vision are diseases that are common in old age: age-related maculopathy, cataract, glaucoma, diabetic retinopathy, and optic nerve atrophy. Almost 10 percent of the population 75 to 84 years of age experiences low vision, while 25 percent of the population 85 and older is deemed to have low vision. Yet, low vision is not confined to the old; an estimated 1 million persons below age 65 experience low vision, and 72 thousand under 65 are blind (Genensky, 1994). An additional 9 million Americans live with other, milder forms of visual impairment that interfere with daily living tasks, especially in adverse lighting conditions (Benson and Marano, 1994).

An important aspect of a person's full participation in today's society is being able to conveniently and confidentially exchange currency in everyday transactions, as when using public transportation or making purchases (EBU, 1994). U.S. citizens with low vision experience a uniquely difficult task in that U.S. banknotes are remarkably uniform in size, color, and general design. The banknotes provide no basis for denominating by blind persons. Visual identification of denomination by people with low vision is generally so challenging that many revert to techniques used by people who are blind.

Blind people must trust others to inform them about the denominations of bills received. In the absence of features that are usable by blind people in the present bills, different denominations, once identified by a trusted sighted person, are sorted and stored in different ways.

FEATURES IN USE WORLDWIDE

The committee has identified 171 issuing authorities in the world producing banknotes. Many have specifically addressed the problems of people with low vision by incorporating such

[1] There are a variety of ways to define levels of visual acuity. One common definition is to find the smallest letters a person can read at a standard distance (traditionally, 20 feet) and express the result as the ratio of this distance to the distance at which a "normal" observer can read the same letters. (In the case cited, the "normal" observer could read the specified letters at 70 feet, hence, acuity of 20/70.)

features as variable size, variable color, and tactile markings. In some cases, a device is made available to blind people to aid in denominating banknotes. For example, England issues a size template, and Canada supplies its blind citizens with a portable banknote reader with audio output.

NEW BANKNOTE DESIGN

By 1996, the U.S. Treasury Department's Bureau of Engraving and Printing (BEP) expects to begin production of a new design for the $100 bill. In each succeeding year, working in descending order, a new design for a denomination will be introduced. By the year 2001, all six denominations currently in production ($100, $50, $20, $10, $5, and $1) will have been redesigned. A major motivation for this redesign is the incorporation of new security features to combat the threat of counterfeiting posed by the rapid development in advanced copying and imaging systems that allow even the unskilled user to make faithful full-color reproductions of documents.

This redesign presents an opportunity to introduce features into the design that will make U.S. banknotes more readily usable by visually disabled people. The timetable of the redesign also presents the opportunity to incorporate features that may require some development work into the smaller denominations within the current redesign sequence. To this end, the Committee on Currency Features Usable by the Visually Impaired was charged to:

- assess features that could be used by people who are visually disabled to recognize, denominate, and authenticate banknotes;
- recommend features that could reasonably be incorporated into banknotes using available technology;
- suggest strategies that should be instituted to make the recommended features most effective; and
- identify research needs in particularly promising areas that could lead to attractive future approaches.

In the study, three aspects of currency transactions were defined: recognition (is this meant to be a banknote?), denomination (how much is it worth?), and authentication (is it a real banknote?). An additional consideration of importance, especially with regard to the use of machines accepting cash, was the usefulness of features indicating orientation of the banknote. The primary goal of the committee was to recommend features that will help visually disabled people denominate banknotes, since reliable denomination is essential to their maintaining independence. The committee also evaluated features that will help these individuals authenticate banknotes, a process for which the individuals have the same needs as the normally sighted public. Such features could be added in addition to those included for use in denomination. The committee did not consider the entire mix of the circulating medium in the U.S. but focused solely on solutions to problems dealing with banknotes.

FEATURE ASSESSMENT CONSIDERATIONS

Over the course of this study, the committee solicited presentations from experts in visual and tactile perception and from representatives of organizations of blind people and people with low vision. The committee also obtained considerable data on currency features usable by visually disabled people and incorporated in the currency of other countries.

The committee generated an extensive list of features representing a wide range of sensory phenomena and application technologies. In assessing and prioritizing these features, the committee used an approach similar to that taken for the evaluation of counterfeit-deterrent features for currency in a previous study (NRC, 1993). In this approach, the set of requirements for a feature was converted into indicators or criteria that were considered in terms of relative importance. The application of the feature to different target populations was considered. Features of use to the broadest range of people were ranked highest.

The criteria for banknote feature effectiveness were first divided into target and evaluation criteria. The target population categories were blind, low vision, normally sighted in adverse lighting, and normally sighted in normal lighting. While visually disabled people were the primary group to be considered in regard to the features, normally sighted people would also benefit from any features implemented. The target function categories were recognition, denomination, authentication, and orientation. Orientation, though significant for use of ATMs (automated teller machines) and vending machines, was given lesser weight.

To evaluate feature effectiveness, technical evaluation criteria that were considered included reliability of readings, ease of use, device requirement, applicability to current bills, compatibility with proposed or existing overt security features, ability to cocirculate with current bills, and resistance to simulation. The unit cost of production, capital costs for the BEP and Federal Reserve banks, effects on note durability, feature survivability, availability for immediate or near-term implementation, and experience as proven banknote technology were considered as implementation evaluation criteria. The possibility of incorporation of a feature in the longer term with some additional development or research was also considered.

Further criteria were used for features that required the use of a device. Device criteria included the ability to recognize and denominate banknotes; accuracy, that is, the number of false positives and false negatives; portability; size; maintenance; cost; response time; power use; and longevity. Ability to authenticate was considered to be an important aspect of future development of devices. The output characteristics for devices should consider potential usage by non-English speakers and should take audible (multilingual), tactile, or visual form. Such devices might find application as point-of-sale aids for cash-accepting machines, which would reduce their unit cost.

COMMITTEE FINDINGS

The committee identified three features useful to visually disabled people that can be incorporated in U.S. banknotes without significant further research: banknote size that differs with denomination, large numerals indicating denomination, and banknote color that differs with banknote denomination. The committee received strong support from representatives of organizations of and for visually disabled people for all three of these features. These features are all used in some form in currencies of other countries, and the technology for production is available today.

Because of the status of the ongoing redesign of the U.S. banknotes, the committee is concerned that features not included in the current redesign will not be implemented until a following redesign. The current design sequence will be complete with the issue of the redesigned bill of the smallest denomination in 2001.

Recommended Features Available Now

To ease denomination of U.S. banknotes, the committee recommends the following features (presented in the order in which they are described in the text, with no priority implied):

- *Banknote size as a key to denomination.* Variation of both length and height would allow for more reliable absolute judgment about denomination, while variation of a single dimension would require a secondary cue, such as a size template, to achieve the same level of reliability.
- *Large, high-contrast numerals on a uniform background.* A large, open space will be required in the banknote design to allow for at least a single numeral, in a plain font, that is larger than one-half the current banknote height.
- *Different predominant colors for each of the six denominations printed.* A single color should dominate at least one face of the banknote and should be sufficiently distinguishable from the other colors in the banknote sequence to remain identifiable even in low lighting.
- *Overt features that could lead to the development of effective, low-cost devices for examining banknotes.* Inclusion of a denomination code is recommended to provide for development of devices for those who have difficulty using the recommended features and to add to the ability of visually disabled people to authenticate banknotes.

Findings and Issues Regarding Recommended Features

- All three of these features will serve the majority of the visually disabled—those with low vision. However, of the three features identified, banknote size that differs with denomination is the only one applicable to the needs of blind people.
- Large numerals and color, if applied in a distinct area, may also be used to indicate banknote orientation. No orientation information is given by different-sized banknotes.
- The Treasury Department should evaluate current approaches and conduct studies to determine the sizing needs of each denomination if the six denominations are to be sufficiently distinguishable. This may require, for instance, starting the sequence with a larger $100 banknote.
- The Treasury Department and the Federal Reserve should identify issues regarding the infrastructure of cash-handling machines to determine an appropriate timetable for the introduction of size-denominated banknotes.

- Development of features building on the substantial literature on visual and tactile processes and perception is warranted for near-term feature additions to banknotes. Highly directed, psychophysical/empirical technical work that addresses questions regarding optimum dimensions, optical contrast, location, colors, physical size, etc., for banknote applications should be undertaken.
- Specification of new or enhanced features should not be aimed at minimal levels of recognition performance (i.e., threshold levels) but should strive for sufficient differentiation to permit rapid, relatively effortless performance, with differences between denominations designed to be several times greater than the difference threshold.
- The committee recommends that research be performed to identify combinations of features that enhance denomination and orientation and, perhaps, authentication.
- In reviewing the needs of the 3.7 million U.S. citizens with low vision, the committee observed that many documents issued by government agencies, such as passports, visas, postage stamps, and food stamps, could better serve those with low vision if features similar to those discussed in the report were incorporated in their design. Indeed, in some cases, features not considered sufficiently robust for application in banknote design might find early application in other government documents.
- The public education campaign accompanying any introduction of new banknote features for visually disabled people would provide a good opportunity for the private sector to consider these types of features for packaging design and related applications.

Recommended Features Requiring Some Additional Research and Development

- The committee urges research on the development of durable tactile features, such as ones printed with "transparent" ink. Transparent-ink tactile marks can be implemented with minimal design changes and so offer flexibility in timing the feature's incorporation.
- The committee recommends research into the implementation issues of holes to denominate banknotes, including the production of durable holes and the psychological questions regarding issuing and using banknotes containing holes.

Research and Development Opportunities

- The committee recommends research to define the threshold and accuracy of reading for the types of low-relief tactile features that are likely to be applicable to banknotes.
- The committee recommends research in the area of enhanced threads, planchettes, or films that would improve devices for examining banknotes.
- The committee recommends that long-term research into advanced features be initiated as possible directions become evident from technology development.
- The committee recommends that analysis regarding the incorporation of advances in microelectronics, nanotechnology, molecular electronics, materials, photonics, and magnetics in device development be an ongoing effort. Research and development efforts directed toward

deriving very sophisticated but inexpensive, reliable, accurate, and inconspicuous devices should be encouraged.

- The BEP should follow the technical work underway by organizations and institutions concerned with the problems of people who are visually disabled and their proposed solutions to those problems, and it should develop a process to assess the applicability of progress in these areas to banknote production.

Implementation Strategies

If the features incorporated in a new design are to be maximally effective, a carefully planned implementation strategy must be developed as the features are evaluated and considered for inclusion. Important aspects of an implementation strategy include the following:

- In selecting features for implementation, the Treasury Department and the Federal Reserve should involve appropriate user groups as early as possible to ensure selection of those features most likely to be used by, and useful to, the target population. The design of any field test should include a cross-section of the target population appropriate to the feature being tested.
- The field test should be broad enough in scope to show not only that the new feature permits recognition under optimal conditions but that rapid, relatively effortless and confidential currency identification are possible across a wide range of everyday circumstances.
- Data gathered from focus groups should be used to help guide the public education campaign that must be a part of the implementation of any new currency feature.
- An appropriate schedule for any introduction of graded sizes of banknotes follows that planned by the BEP for the banknote redesign, beginning with the $100. Since this banknote would be the largest in the series and represents the smallest production volume, gradual introduction of size-denominated banknotes over the course of six to seven years would allow time for the commercial currency handling industry to prepare for the change.
- In the early stages of distributing sized banknotes, templates would have to be made available to visibly disabled people. The templates might be distributed through banks or appropriate organizations of visually disabled people.

REFERENCES

Benson, V., and M.A. Marano. 1994. Current estimates from the National Health Interview Survey. National Center for Health Statistics, January 1994. Vital and Health Statistics Series 10(189):95.

EBU (European Blind Union). 1994. A report of the European Blind Union Expert Working Group on Currency: Recommendations for the Design of the ECU. Paris, France: EBU.

Genensky, S. 1994. Personal communication to the Committee on Currency Features Usable by the Visually Impaired. March 30, 1994.

NRC (National Research Council). 1993. Counterfeit Deterrent Features for the Next-Generation Currency Design. National Materials Advisory Board, NRC. Washington, D.C.: National Academy Press.

1

INTRODUCTION

The currency of the United States of America is the most widely used in the world. The U.S. banknotes that are used today were first produced in 1929, and there have been only minor changes to the basic designs since then. The designs of the six denominations currently in production ($1, $5, $10, $20, $50, and $100)[1] were intended to make it difficult to counterfeit U.S. banknotes by common printing processes, to be durable, and to be a means of differentiating each denomination. U.S. paper currency differs from the currency of all other countries in that notes of all denominations are of identical size and color. To ensure that the correct denomination is being given and that the correct amount of change is received in return, extra care is required of a person using a bill.

Features that may be used in future banknote designs to authenticate U.S. banknotes were recommended in a previous report (NRC, 1993). On July 13, 1994, the U.S. Department of the Treasury announced its intent to issue redesigned banknotes that incorporate counterfeit-deterrent features, which are based on the recommendations of the National Research Council study and other studies performed by the New Currency Design Task Force. The visible security features scheduled for incorporation in the new design are described in Appendix F.

Since all the U.S. banknotes are the same size (approximately 67 mm × 156 mm) and are printed with identical inks on the same security paper, the user has to refer to the printed design to determine the denomination of the banknote. On each of the six denominations in production today, centered on the banknote front there is a portrait unique to that denomination note. The value of the note is printed in grey letters (1.6 cm high) across the green Treasury seal and in smaller, black letters (3–4 mm in height) across the bottom center of both the front and the back of the note. The denomination numeral is printed in all four corners of the note on both front and back, with the exception of the $5 bill, which has the word "FIVE" in place of the numerals on the lower part of the back side. The backs of these banknotes are generally more distinctive than the fronts, with a picture of a different building on each (except the $1 bill, which shows the obverse and reverse of the Great Seal of the United States, and the $2 bill, which shows the signing of the Declaration of Independence). Each denomination note also has characteristic intricately engraved scrollwork around the borders of the front and back of the note. In addition

---

[1] Although still legal tender, the $2 banknote is currently not in regular production. No decision regarding issuance of this note in the new design series has been made.

to these features found on U.S. banknotes of all denominations, some of the designs include additional value and numeral indicators, such as the word "TEN" printed through the numerals on the back of the $10 bill. In general, the additional features are printed in smaller fonts than the more prominent denominators on the top of the banknote face.

For cash transactions, all of the features present in the design either to help the user verify the legitimacy of a particular banknote or to indicate its value are visual clues, with the exception of the characteristic "feel" of U.S. banknotes. For blind people or those with low vision,[2] distinguishing among bills of different denominations and determining the authenticity of a bill can be difficult or impossible. Approximately 3.5 million Americans have low vision, which is defined as any form of visual disability not correctable with glasses or contact lenses that affects everyday activities. And nearly 200,000 additional Americans are blind—that is, they have no useful pattern vision. For these groups, the current banknote design causes problems in the daily activities of buying and selling merchandise, using vending machines, and generally working with money. For many other Americans, dealing with money in lighting that is less than ideal can also lead to errors in cash transactions.

The currency designs of other countries attempt to address the problems of blind people and those with low vision by identifying the value of a banknote with a variety of features (see Appendix D). A common technique is to make bills of different values different sizes. Using a size template or, with some practice, by feel, a blind person can differentiate among bills of various denominations by size alone. The use of different colors for different denominations is also common in currency outside the United States and is of use to many with low vision. Appendix D contains descriptions of several additional features in use worldwide that help visually disabled people to more easily effect cash transactions.

Within the United States, there is a long history of groups advocating changes to the U.S. banknotes to make them more user-friendly. For example, the American Council of the Blind has adopted resolutions over the last 20 years to encourage the Bureau of Engraving and Printing (BEP) to investigate and adopt features to make banknote denomination possible for blind people (ACB, 1972, 1977, 1978, 1979, 1980, 1992). In the early 1960s, the BEP invited people who were blind and visually impaired to provide comments about identifying U.S. currency (Hill, 1994). From the 1970s to the 1990s, several resolutions were introduced in Congress to urge the Secretary of the Treasury and the BEP to provide braille markings and tactile markings on banknotes for currency identification (H.R., 1979, 1981, 1983a, b, 1991; S., 1983).

In 1983, the BEP, in conjunction with the Federal Reserve and the Secret Service, conducted a study into worldwide efforts to make currency accessible to blind people and those with low vision. They concluded that making banknote size proportional to the denomination would be the most effective way to ease identification of a banknote's value. The report suggested that there would be a high cost associated with radical redesign of the U.S. banknotes. In that report, delivered to Representative Edward Roybal (then Chairman of the Select Committee on Aging, U.S. House of Representatives), the BEP recommended the continuing development of sophisticated electronic devices to determine the denomination of a banknote and provide either an audio or tactile output. Due to current efforts to redesign the U.S. banknotes,

---

[2]There are varying definitions for these terms. See the glossary (Appendix C) and discussion in Chapter 2 for the definitions used by the committee throughout this report.

the present study was conducted without the constraint of leaving the U.S. banknote design intact.

Features currently used by other countries, and others previously proposed by groups representing blind and visually impaired people in the United States (for example, ACB, 1978, 1980, 1992), can be considered for inclusion in the forthcoming redesign of U.S. currency without compromising the security of American banknotes. This report contains an analysis by the Committee on Currency Features Usable by Visually Impaired of the problems encountered by people with visual disabilities when dealing with U.S. paper money and it contains recommended solutions to those problems. In Chapter 2, the populations of visually disabled people are described, and their needs in working with currency are assessed. Chapter 3 contains a description of the assessment methodology undertaken by the committee in evaluating various proposed banknote features, followed by the assessment of the individual features and recommendations in Chapter 4. Chapter 5 contains recommendations for research and development in areas of particular promise. And Chapter 6 presents strategies for implementing the features recommended. Throughout the report, a series of recommendations are made; these are compiled in Chapter 7.

REFERENCES

ACB (American Council of the Blind). 1972. Resolution 72-08. Approved July 7, 1972.

ACB (American Council of the Blind). 1977. Resolution 77-07. Approved July 16, 1977.

ACB (American Council of the Blind). 1978. Resolution 78-24. Approved July 29, 1978.

ACB (American Council of the Blind). 1979. Resolution 79-23. Approved July 7, 1979.

ACB (American Council of the Blind). 1980. Resolution 80-04. Approved July 7, 1980.

ACB (American Council of the Blind). 1992. Resolution 92-02. Approved July 9, 1992.

Hill, B. J. 1994. Presentation to the Committee by Billie Jean Hill on behalf of the Council of Citizens with Low Vision. March 29, 1994.

H.R. (U.S. House of Representatives). 1979. House Congressional Resolution 6027. Introduced December 4, 1979, to the House Committee on Banking, Finance and Urban Affairs.

H.R. (U.S. House of Representatives). 1981. House Congressional Resolution 3656. Introduced May 20, 1981, to the House Committee on Banking, Finance and Urban Affairs.

H.R. (U.S. House of Representatives). 1983a. House Congressional Resolution 2666. Introduced April 20, 1983, to the House Committee on Banking, Finance and Urban Affairs.

H.R. (U.S. House of Representatives). 1983b. House Congressional Resolution 163. Introduced September 13, 1983, to the House Committee on Banking, Finance and Urban Affairs.

H.R. (U.S. House of Representatives). 1991. House Congressional Resolution 2160. Introduced May 1, 1991, to the House Committee on Banking, Finance and Urban Affairs.

NRC (National Research Council). 1993. Counterfeit Deterrent Features for the Next-Generation Currency Design. National Materials Advisory Board, NRC. Washington, D.C.: National Academy Press.

S. (U.S. Senate). 1983. Senate Congressional Resolution 1877. Introduced September 22, 1983, to the Senate Committee on Banking, Housing and Urban Affairs.

2

DEFINITION OF NEEDS AND STATEMENT OF REQUIREMENTS

As discussed in the Introduction, the United States is alone in issuing paper currency bills in which all denominations are of identical size and color. The numbers on the corners of the bills are small and of low contrast, making them difficult to read by people with impaired vision. For everyday transactions, U.S. paper currency possesses no nonvisual identifying features, rendering it impossible for blind people to denominate bills without assistance. The lack of distinctive visual features and the total absence of nonvisual features for the common user constitute a hindrance to commerce and daily living for millions of visually disabled people. In addition, the lack of distinctive features results in problems of denomination for a much wider population with mild visual impairments, including those impairments acquired during the normal aging process, and for anyone in a poorly lit environment.

The goal of this report is to recommend features for inclusion in U.S. banknotes that will enhance denomination and authentication of bills by the entire population. Because currency transactions occur every day and are critical to full participation in society, it is essential that the currency be usable by everyone. Currency identification should be "user friendly," that is, it should be effective across the widest possible range of circumstances.

In this chapter, the committee describes the affected population and the practical nature and extent of the problem. The specific needs for currency identification among subgroups of the affected populations are outlined, along with existing solutions. Requirements that should be satisfied by future improvements to the banknotes are indicated.

From the user's point of view, key objectives of currency identification include accuracy, speed, and confidentiality across a wide range of lighting conditions and for both new and worn banknotes. Under all conditions, users would like to have fast and nearly effortless transactions; features that slow down transactions, such as the need for specialized equipment, or features that require extended effort of scrutiny or comparison run counter to this objective. In addition, users want to identify currency independently with their own senses (possibly assisted by such everyday aids as eyeglasses or hearing aids).

A benchmark of effectiveness for new features is to make banknotes as identifiable as coinage. U.S. coins can be identified rapidly, effortlessly, and independently by almost everyone, in a wide range of conditions. Coins do this by using a combination of features that include graduated size, weight, color (base material), and textured edges; they thus are identifiable by touch and by vision.

TARGET POPULATION

Many terms have been used to refer to visual impairment. For consistency, the committee will rely primarily on "visual disability," "low vision," "blindness," and "mild visual impairment" as defined below and in the glossary.[1]

It has been estimated by the National Advisory Eye Council (1993) that there are more than three million people in the United States who are visually disabled. "Visually disabled" refers to those who are blind or have low vision. There are approximately 200,000 people who are blind; they have no useful pattern vision, but some may retain light perception. The remaining people in the visually disabled category have low vision. Low vision is often defined as best-corrected letter acuity less than 20/60 in the better eye (World Health Organization, 1966) or the inability to read regular newsprint with optimal reading glasses.[2] Some people with severe peripheral-field loss are classified as having low vision even though their letter acuity may be higher than the 20/60 criterion. The estimated number of people with low vision and blindness in the United States divided by age group is given in Table 2-1 and is also shown in Figure 2-1.[3] The data in this table were generated by applying the data analysis technique explained in Genensky (1978) to the 1990 U.S. Census data (Genensky, 1994). According to these data, there are approximately 3.7 visually disabled Americans.

The leading causes of low vision and blindness are diseases that are common in old age: age-related maculopathy, cataract, glaucoma, diabetic retinopathy, and optic nerve atrophy. According to data from the Health Interview Survey, more than two-thirds of all people with low vision are 65 years of age or older, coming to an estimated total of 2.9 million people in 1990 (Nelson and Dimitrova, 1993). It is estimated that more than 25 percent of all people over 85 years of age are visually disabled (Genensky, 1994). As the geriatric population grows, the number of people with low vision and other age-related disabilities will increase.

The two traditional clinical measures of low vision are acuity and visual field. A recent detailed discussion of the measurement of visual acuity and visual field has been provided by the National Research Council Committee on Vision (NRC, 1994).

---

[1] "Legal blindness" is commonly defined as a visual acuity in the better eye (with best refractive correction) of no more than 20/200 or a visual field of no more than 20 degrees. Approximately 600,000–900,000 persons in the United States fall into this category, which is primarily used for legal and official purposes. Visual disability and visual impairment encompass a broader population than legal blindness; blindness encompasses a narrower population.

[2] The level of best-corrected visual acuity at which a person is said to have "low vision" has several definitions. Measured levels of 20/60 or 20/70 are commonly used and correspond roughly to the more qualitative definition of inability to read regular newsprint. The definition used by each source of the data cited in the chapter is given with that data.

[3] Because the braille print version of this report will not contain the graphics, each figure is described in detail in the text.

Table 2-1 Estimated 1990 U.S. Population with Low Vision and Blindness by Age Category, as Number of People and as Percentage of the Age Group Population [a]

Age	Estimated Number of People			Percentage of Age Group	
	Low Vision[b]	Blind[c]	U.S. Population	Low Vision[b]	Blind[c]
0 - 4	6,200	800	18,354,400	0.03	0.004
5 - 19	117,200	12,200	53,067,900	0.22	0.02
20 - 44	390,600	29,100	99,674,700	0.39	0.03
45 - 64	463,600	30,300	46,371,000	1.00	0.07
65 - 74	805,400	28,200	18,106,600	4.45	0.16
75 - 84	964,700	48,600	10,055,100	9.59	0.48
85 & older	775,800	37,700	3,080,200	25.19	1.22
total	3,523,500	186,900	248,709,800	1.42	0.08

Source: Genensky, 1978, 1994.

[a] Data concerning persons 0–64 years old were analyzed by S. Genensky, and data concerning persons 65 years old or older were analyzed by C. Kirchner.

[b] "Low vision" for this table is defined as corrected visual acuity of no better than 20/70 in the better eye or a maximum diameter of visual field of no more than 30 degrees. The low-vision category does not include blind individuals.

[c] "Blind" for this table and this report refers to persons with no useful pattern vision, who are referred to as "functionally blind" in the original reference.

Acuity is measured by finding the smallest letters a person can read at a standard distance (traditionally, 20 feet) and expressing the result as the ratio of this distance to the distance at which a "normal" observer can read the same letters. For example, a person with 20/60 can just read letters at 20 feet that a person with 20/20 acuity can read at 60 feet. People with low vision have acuities ranging from less than 20/60 to 20/2000. The denominator of the fraction in visual acuity notation can also be thought of as the letter size. This size is defined as the distance at which the observer must stand for the letter to subtend an angle of 5 minutes of arc. For example, a letter size indicating 20/20 visual acuity is equivalent to 5 minutes of arc; 20/200 to 50 minutes; etc.

Feature size, viewing distance, and the user's acuity put boundary conditions on the identification of banknotes. The large corner digits on the portrait side of $1 and $10 U.S.

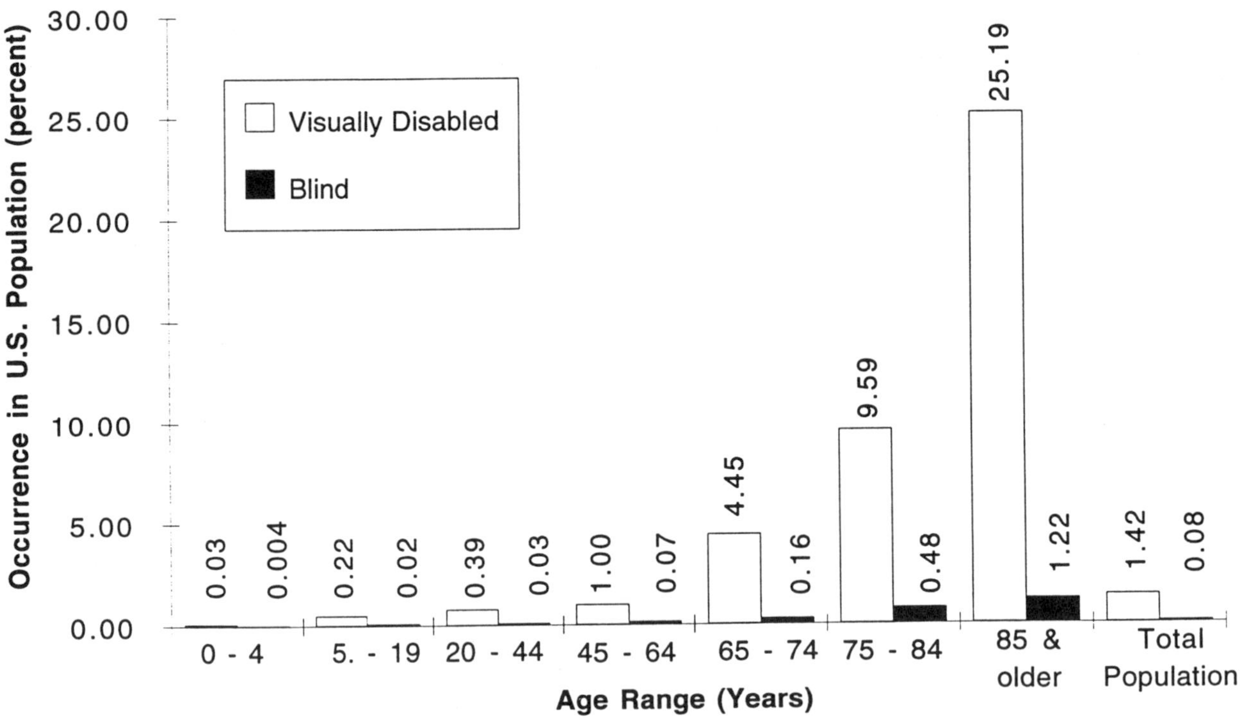

Figure 2-1 Percentage by age group of 1990 U.S. population with visual disabilities.

banknotes would be at the visual limit for someone with 20/400 letter acuity, if they were viewed at a normal reading distance of 16 inches (40 cm). Suppose the viewing distance is increased to 40 inches (1 m), roughly the distance from the eye to a bill on a checkout counter. The corner digits would now be at or beyond the acuity limit of people with about 20/160 vision. Identification at the acuity limit is slow and requires optimal viewing conditions, including good lighting and 100 percent black/white numeral contrast, which is not true even of crisp, new currency bills. Conservatively, symbols should be at least a factor of two larger than the acuity limit for practical use. Only people with acuity better than about 20/80 would meet this more stringent "factor of two" criterion for viewing the currency digits on a bill on the counter. Following this informal argument, most people with low vision (acuity less than 20/60) experience difficulty recognizing the large digits on present banknotes in a common cash transaction.

It should be noted that clinical definitions of acuity are based on controlled tests conducted under ideal viewing conditions—bold black letters on a pure white background (near 100 percent contrast), good illumination, no distracting symbols, and no time pressure. By comparison, the letters and numbers on U.S. money bills are of much lower contrast (discussed later in this chapter), are closely surrounded by distracting abstract designs, and are often viewed under low illumination with little time for prolonged scrutiny. As a result, direct extrapolation from acuity testing to feature recognition on bills is likely to underestimate the number of people who will experience difficulty.

Visual-field size refers to the range of visual directions, centered on the line of sight, over which a standardized test target can be detected. Field loss results from damage to portions of the retina, resulting in blind regions in the visual field. The various scenarios shown in Figure 2-2 illustrate the effects of different types of visual-field loss and are discussed in detail below.

Age-related macular degeneration (AMD) afflicts many older people and is the leading cause of low vision. Because vision is lost in the high-resolution central portion of the visual field, afflicted individuals must rely on sight in their low-resolution peripheral vision. Figure 2-2 shows the same photo of New York City's Metropolitan Opera House a number of times—once in sharp focus (Figure 2-2a) and then as it would be seen with various types of visual impairment (figures 2-2b through 2-2e). Figure 2-2b shows the picture with the central field completely blocked, illustrating a severe case of age-related macular degeneration. Typically, reading is impaired, and individuals afflicted with this degeneration require large letters (high magnification) to read.

Some diseases, such as advanced glaucoma or retinitis pigmentosa, can result in the loss of almost all peripheral vision. Only a small island of central vision remains (tunnel vision). Figure 2-2c illustrates vision with this type of impairment. Individuals with this form of low vision may have fairly high acuity, but they experience great difficulty in mobility (walking or driving), and they have problems in visual search tasks (e.g., finding signs, page numbers, or currency digits). Other diseases, such as diabetic retinopathy, can result in patchy vision with losses in a number of areas within the visual field, as illustrated in Figure 2-2d. Since it is impossible to accurately portray what vision loss is like for a person with low vision, the illustrations in these figures are meant only to demonstrate the types of vision loss that *might* occur with various diseases and impairments. However, it should be remembered that the scotomatous (blind) areas in these simulations would move with the eye, so, for example, a person with age-related macular degeneration will *always* have a centrally located blind spot when viewing different areas of the picture.

In addition to low acuity and reduced field, a third kind of visual deficit, intensively studied in recent years, is reduced contrast sensitivity (see illustration in Figure 2-2e). Figure 2-3 demonstrates the effects of this type of visual impairment; imagine reading text printed with contrasts of 60 percent ("he made plans"), 30 percent ("to go camping"), 13 percent ("and hiking in"), and 6.5 percent ("the mountains"). Many types of eye disease, such as cataract, can cause a reduction in retinal-image contrast or a loss of sensitivity to contrast by retinal neurons. The consequence is an effective reduction in the contrast (difference between light and dark areas) of images. People with normal vision have a substantial tolerance to contrast reduction for many visual tasks. In the case of reading, print contrast can be quite low (down to 10 percent) before there is much effect on reading speed (Legge et al., 1987). For many people with low vision, however, and for those with normal aging vision, there is much less tolerance to poor contrast. For such people, even rather small reductions in print contrast can adversely affect reading (Rubin and Legge, 1989).

Two aspects of contrast are relevant to currency design. Contrast polarity specifies whether the letters are light and the background dark, or vice versa. The contrast polarity of

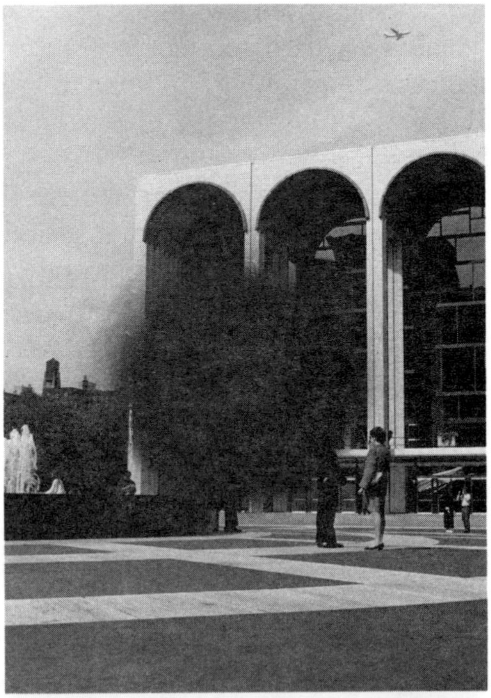

b

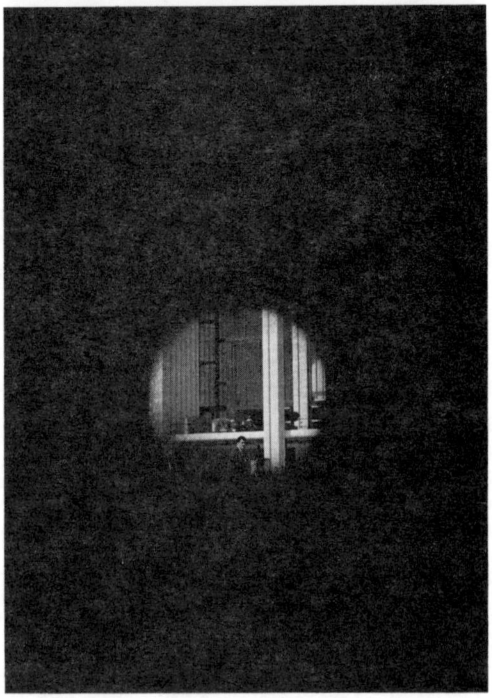

c

Figure 2-2 Illustrations of various types of visual impairment using photos of New York's Metropolitan Opera House: (a) normal vision; (b) central field loss; (c) peripheral field loss; (d) patchy vision loss; (e) reduced contrast. Source: The Jewish Guild for the Blind, 1992.

alphanumeric symbols usually has little effect on recognition for people with normal vision. For some people with low vision (especially those with ocular light scatter due to cataracts), acuity and reading performance are better for the light-on-dark polarity, which is a property of present U.S. banknotes.

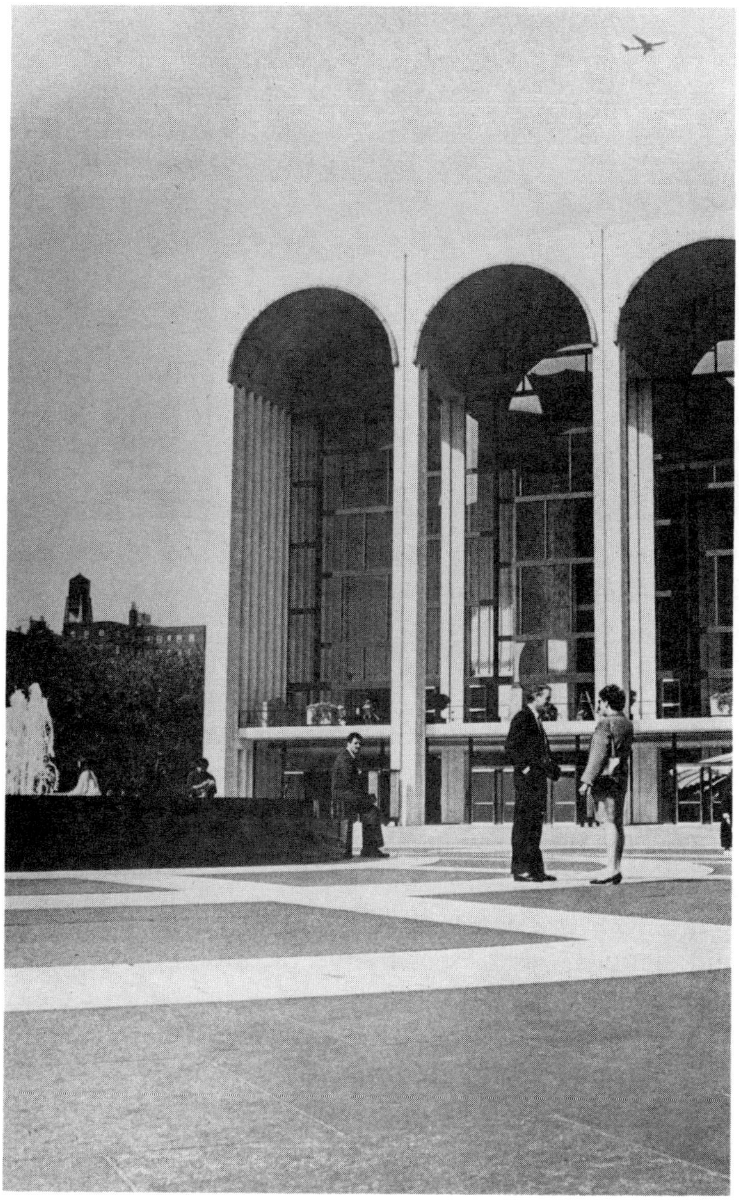

a

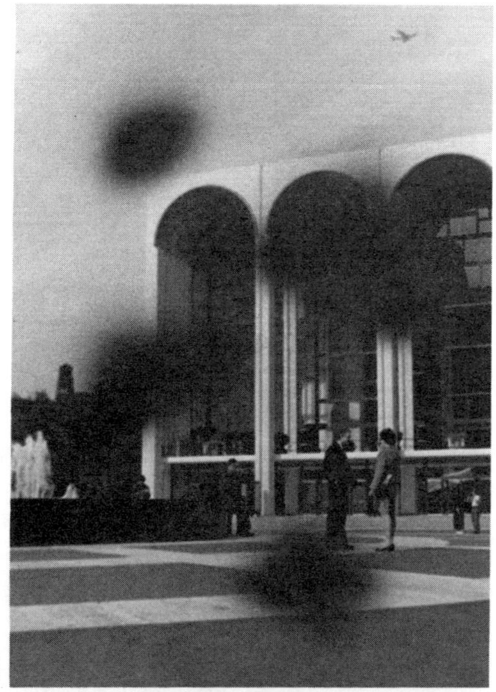

d

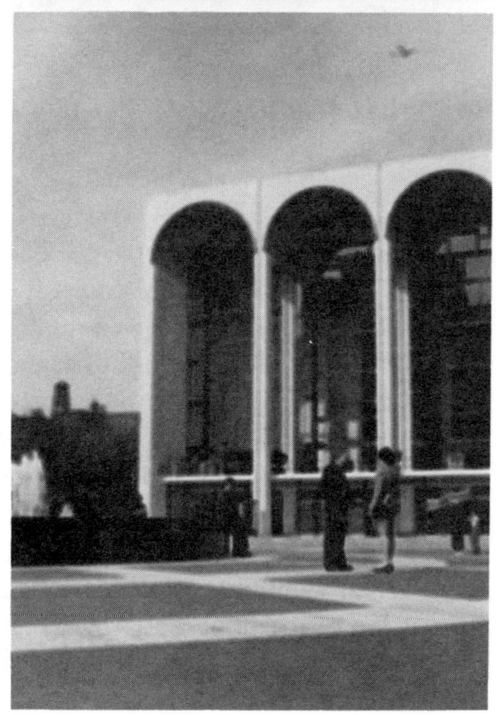

e

More important than polarity is the overall contrast level. Photometric measurements by a member of the committee of the contrast of the large corner digits on the portrait side of $1

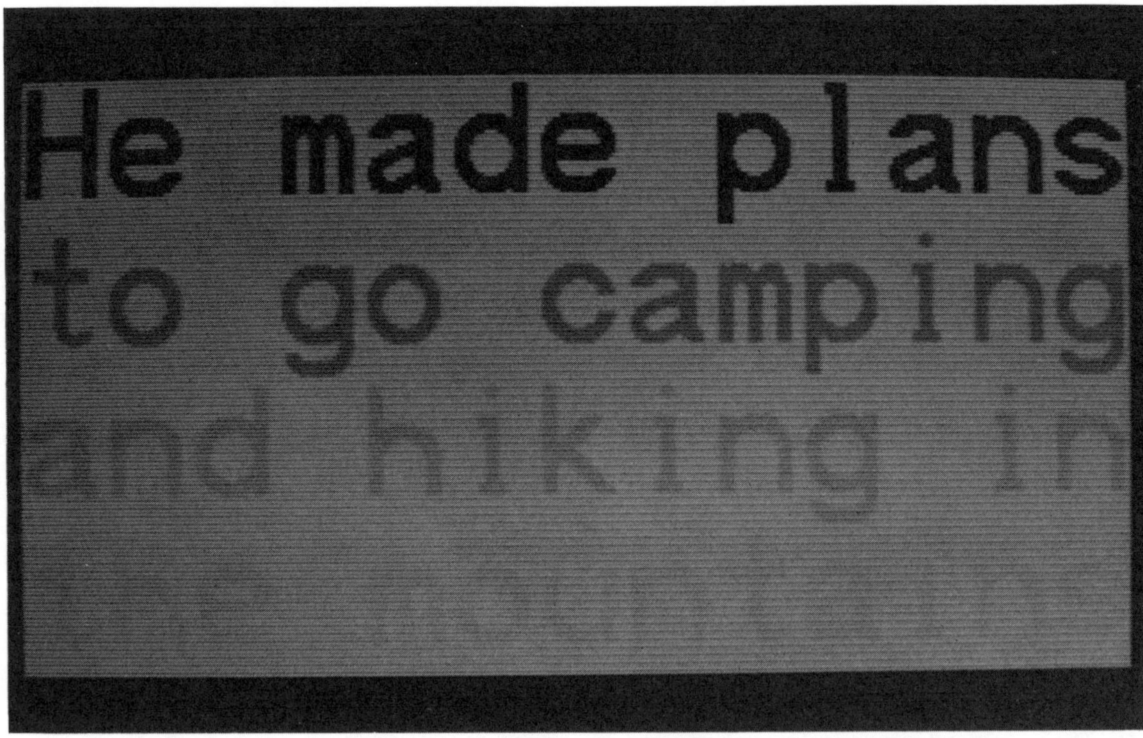

Figure 2-3 Lines of text in decreasing contrast demonstrating visual effects of loss of contrast sensitivity. Reprinted from Legge, 1993, courtesy of Massachusetts Institute of Technology Press.

notes indicated contrasts of 60 percent (new crisp bill) and 30 percent (worn bill).[4] The reduction from 100 percent contrast undoubtedly has an adverse effect on recognition for many people with low vision, even under optimal viewing conditions. Under conditions of poor visibility (especially low lighting and long viewing distance), the suboptimal contrast will also take its toll on recognition by normally sighted people.

In addition to the 3.7 million visually disabled Americans, there are many people with mild visual impairment due to peripheral field deficits, glare sensitivity, or losses in contrast sensitivity. Estimates of the number of Americans with mild forms of visual impairment, referred to here as visually impaired, extend to nearly 9 million (Benson and Marano, 1994).

When viewing conditions are bad (often the case for poorly lit indoor settings or at night), the portion of the population likely to have difficulty identifying U.S. banknotes is much larger. Under poor lighting conditions, the visual acuity of persons with "normal" vision is compromised, while the visual capabilities of those with mild visual impairments due to disease or the natural cause of aging are further reduced.

Even in the absence of disease, aging eyes are particularly disadvantaged in recognition tasks in poor illumination. For example, the reduced pupil size of an average 80-year-old

---

[4] Contrast is defined as $100*(L_{max} - L_{min})/(L_{max} + L_{min})$ where L_{max} is the luminance of the digit, and L_{min} is the luminance of the background of the digit.

compared with that of a 20-year-old will allow only one-quarter as much light to enter the eye (Pitts, 1982). This diminished light is then diffused and scattered by opacities in the optical media (which increase with age) before it reaches the retina, which is likely to be reduced in its ability to detect low contrast features. The net result is a severe reduction in visual performance under adverse lighting conditions for older people.

The committee notes also that special difficulties are encountered by individuals with multiple disabilities. New currency features relying on sound would not be accessible to people who are both hearing and visually disabled, for example, the 10,000 individuals with Usher syndrome in the United States (RPFFB, 1994). Also, individuals with decreased tactile sensitivity accompanying visual impairment (e.g., from diabetes) may not benefit from subtle tactile features (Cholewiak, 1994).

It is important to note that normally sighted Americans would clearly benefit in ease of use, especially in conditions of adverse visibility, from most features intended for use by visually disabled people.

Some who are working for the full integration of blind people in American society have expressed opposition to certain special features (such as obvious "braille" markings), for fear that these markings would be a ubiquitous signal that special accommodations are required for blind people (Maurer, 1994). The committee evaluated prospective features with respect to their ability to enhance the recognition of the currency by all users.

CURRENCY IDENTIFICATION NEEDS

The currency identification needs of our target population can be conveniently divided into commercial and daily-living categories. A commercial need for currency identification arises for those who are engaged in any kind of retail or other trade in which ability to identify currency is a necessary part of the job. Lack of suitable banknote identification features raises obstacles to employment in such jobs. Daily activities include using currency in many situations, such as purchasing groceries and using public transportation.

Significant experience and insight comes from visually disabled workers who operate cafeterias or vending stands, usually in government-owned buildings, under the Randolph Sheppard Act Business Enterprises Program. In 1992, there were almost 3,500 people employed under this program, doing more than $395 million in business (Abbott, 1994; RSVFP, 1993). Such workers must accept bills rapidly and give out accurate change as a routine part of the job. A blind cashier cannot independently identify bills in a transaction and must rely on the customer.[5] This arrangement may result in fraud or costly mistakes.

Visually disabled people face problems in identifying U.S. banknotes in broader daily living situations. For blind individuals, the overwhelming need is for denomination without dependence on a sighted person. For people with low vision, needs vary according to the nature

---

[5] There are anecdotal stories that some blind people are able to denominate U.S. currency without any artificial aid. Although some people who are "legally blind" have sufficient vision to identify bills, the committee was unable to substantiate through literature search or interaction with representatives of associations of blind people any such claims for people who are blind.

of the visual deficit and the ambient lighting conditions as discussed earlier in this chapter. An older person with macular degeneration may have relatively little difficulty in identifying bills at a well lit checkout counter but may be unable to identify bills in a dimly lit restaurant or in a taxi at night.

Although denomination of banknotes is the committee's primary focus, it is frequently useful to know the orientation of a bill. Specific orientation of bills is required by some money-changing machines and for stacking purposes by banks. A currency feature that conveys bill orientation would be useful for such purposes.

In both commercial and daily-living situations, successful currency transactions require rapid and accurate denomination of banknotes without the need for lengthy inspection or thought. To achieve this goal, specification of new or enhanced features should not be aimed at minimal levels of recognition performance (i.e., threshold levels) but should strive for sufficient differentiation to permit rapid, effortless performance. For example, research on reading has shown that letter sizes should be three to five times larger than acuity values in order to achieve comfortable and rapid reading (Legge, 1991). Similar consideration should be applied to currency identification features.

DISCRIMINATION VERSUS ABSOLUTE JUDGMENT

This chapter has focused on the difficulties encountered by visually disabled people in currency identification. The design of new visual, tactile, or other features for banknote identification should take into consideration perceptual limitations on discrimination and absolute judgment that limit performance by everyone. The challenge is to design features that can code six denominations of bills ($1, $5, $10, $20, $50, and $100) in a way that circumvents these perceptual limitations.

Discrimination refers to the perceptual ability to compare two physical magnitudes (e.g., weights, light intensities, tonal frequencies, lengths, etc.) and tell them apart. The smallest difference that can be reliably discriminated is called the difference threshold. For perceptual discrimination on many physical dimensions, the difference threshold is constant (or nearly constant) in percentage terms across the range of that dimension. This constancy is termed Weber's Law, and is expressed as:

$$D/D' = k$$

where D is the difference threshold, D' is the physical magnitude, and k is a constant (the Weber fraction). Several examples are shown in Table 2-2. As an example, according to this table, two weights can be discriminated if they differ by more than 4.3 percent. The discrimination of length by the sense of touch alone is a very complicated experimental problem because of the variety of sensory inputs a human being uses when trying to identify an object by touch. It is not clear that this simple form of Weber's law is applicable to the task of distinguishing length by the sense of touch.

Some possible features for coding currency denomination, such as size or roughness, can be analyzed in terms of their difference thresholds. In designing a code:

1. The magnitude of change between denominations should always exceed the difference thresholds.
2. Perceptual discrimination is typically slow when operating near the threshold value. For this reason, it is prudent to have step sizes several times larger than the difference threshold.
3. Assuming Weber's law applies to variations in length, differences between the sizes of successive denominations should probably be constant in percentage terms, not linear terms.
4. For some dimensions, the difference threshold may increase in old age.

Inherent in discrimination is a comparison between two stimuli. In the case of banknote identification, the comparison may be between two bills (based on size, weight, etc.) or between a bill and a measuring gauge.

A second kind of perceptual judgment, called absolute judgment, may be more important to currency identification. Absolute judgment refers to the ability to identify any one of N distinct values along a physical dimension. For example, imagine having N different weights, or N light intensities, or N loudness levels of a given tone, etc. A human subject has to learn to attach labels to these stimuli so they can be identified when presented on their own. Miller

Table 2-2 A Summary of Weber Fractions

Stimulus	Weber Fraction (%)
Intensity of pure tone	20 [a]
Amplitude of vibration	24.5
Frequency of vibration	10
Visual contrast	10 [a]
Hue - red/yellow	0.6
Hue - green/yellow	2.9
Finger span	2.1
Lifted weight	4.3
Luminance	17
Skin pressure	17
Taste - salt	25
Taste - sucrose	17

Data extracted from Laming, 1986.

[a] For these stimuli, the Weber fraction is not constant over the range of stimulus magnitude. The Weber fraction in these cases decreases as the stimulus magnitude increases, indicating that more subtle changes in visual contrast or tone loudness are distinguishable at higher absolute stimulus magnitude.

(1956) summarized many findings on absolute judgment. He showed that when N is 4 or less, people tend to be accurate in absolute judgment. When N rises to about 7 (plus or minus 2), people begin to make errors. There is some variation across stimulus dimensions. The key point is that if banknotes are coded as six points along a single physical dimension (such as length, roughness, thickness), people are likely to make some errors in absolute judgment when a single cue is present. That is, if presented with a single bill (with no measuring gauge or other bill for comparison), some errors are likely to be made. Recognizing that humans are limited to sets of less than seven in their ability to make absolute judgments is a case for limiting the number of denominations of banknotes in general circulation to no more than the present six, and even fewer would be preferable.[6] In the same article, Miller reviewed evidence that accuracy of absolute judgment can be increased if two or more independent dimensions are used to code information. In the context of currency identification, this means that accuracy in identification of six denominations is likely to be improved if two dimensions are used for coding (e.g., length and texture, or length and edge profile as in coinage). This likelihood was confirmed in a demonstration experiment conducted by the committee, which is briefly described in Chapter 4 in connection with the size feature.

To summarize the research into discrimination and absolute judgment: (1) Data on perceptual discrimination can provide lower bounds on the step sizes for coding denomination along a physical dimension. (2) Coding six items (denominations) on a single physical dimension (e.g., length) is likely to result in some errors of absolute judgment. (3) Accuracy can be improved by using two independent dimensions for coding the six items.

EXISTING CURRENCY DENOMINATION TECHNIQUES

Many visually disabled people must trust others to inform them about the denomination of bills received. Once identified, these bills must be sorted for accurate retrieval later. Due to the absence of tactual or other identifying features in the present bills, many blind individuals employ a system of folding to assist in this process. Different denominations, once identified by a trusted sighted person, are folded in different ways (diagonally, crosswise, etc.) according to denomination. Sometimes, people with low vision forego visual identification and revert to techniques used by people who are blind.

Under good lighting conditions, persons with low vision identify bills by holding them close to the eye. An optical magnifier may be necessary for focus. The ease of identification depends on a host of factors, including the level and direction of lighting and the nature of visual impairment.

Machines are available that can denominate and to some extent authenticate banknotes for blind individuals. The smallest of these, costing approximately $400, is 6×3×1 inches in size,

---

[6] The replacement of the current $1 banknote with a $1 coin might be used to reduce the number of banknote denominations, and would be a benefit to visually disabled people for that reason. However, there are a great many other issues surrounding the change to a $1 coin, such as the economic impact, public acceptance, and environmental impact, that the committee was not qualified to address, so the idea is noted here, but is not fully assessed for recommendation.

can be carried in a pocket or purse, and provides a talking output denominating the bill that is inserted. However, the devices are not always reliable, especially on crumpled and dirty bills, and are relatively slow. Audio output in the form of synthetic speech is not usually private, although an earphone can be used if desired. In commercial situations, blind vendors sometimes use nonportable automatic currency identifiers retailing for approximately $900. This device is intended to provide more-reliable authentication abilities than smaller, less expensive devices and provides a series of auditory "beeps" as output, enhancing privacy compared with synthetic speech. It is possible to integrate some of these devices with the cash register. However, reports provided to the committee by a representative of the approximately 3,500 Randolph Sheppard vendors indicated that these machines significantly slow down transactions and are usually bypassed in favor of asking the customer what denomination is handed to the vendor (Abbott, 1994). The devices, as currently available, do not yet fully meet the needs of users for fast and confidential banknote identification. In addition, their bulk and high cost are barriers to widespread use. Development of these devices by groups not associated with the banknote designers (e.g., The American Foundation for the Blind) is limited by their having to determine denomination-distinctive features and patterns around which to design sensors. A major cost of developing these devices is in determining these features and patterns (Schreier, 1994). A discussion of the criteria for an ideal denominating device is contained in Chapter 3.

Existing approaches in other countries (see Appendix D) that can be used by visually disabled people to denominate banknotes include the use of bills of varying sizes and colors. The use of varying sizes reportedly allows a blind individual to denominate bills accurately using a simple, inexpensive plastic guide. With practice, discrimination between various bills can be made without the guide. The use of different sizes also provides a redundant cue for sighted individuals when sorting money bills, allowing, for example, a $1 note to be selected from a group of bills carried inside a pocket without withdrawing the entire group. The ease of using different-sized coins indicates that this method of differentiating value becomes second nature once a person becomes familiar with the size/value correlation.

Most other countries also use different predominant colors for each denomination. The simple detection of color is faster than finding and reading printed numbers, especially for those with poor letter acuity. It should be noted, however, that many people with low vision have difficulty in discriminating subtle shades of color and that color cues are generally less obvious at low levels of illumination. Consequently, any added color features should use clearly distinguishable colors.

Some foreign currencies, including the new series of Canadian notes introduced in 1986, also contain numerals of much larger size and higher contrast than those found on U.S. banknotes to facilitate identification for people with normal and low vision.

There are also several countries using tactile denomination symbols, such as printed bars or shaped grids of small dots, on their banknotes, and visually disabled people in these countries can use these marks to recognize and denominate the banknotes.

USER NEEDS AND REQUIREMENTS

All the user groups discussed require a means of currency denomination that can be summarized briefly as follows:

- The method of denomination ideally should be rapid, easy, and confidential.
- The method should not require special devices or equipment, other than everyday aids such as eyeglasses.

Based on these general user considerations and other considerations of the technical implementation of such features, the committee developed an evaluation system for the different possible banknote features under consideration (see Chapter 3).

SUMMARY

It is clear that a major need exists for a better means of banknote denomination for the 3.7 million Americans with visual disabilities, with the goal of giving this population the full access to currency handling available to the rest of society and to visually disabled people in other countries. In addition, due to the increasing number of older individuals with impaired vision due to minor eye disease or the normal aging process, such features would be of great benefit to a far wider population than that represented by the current statistics on blindness and low vision. Certain new features, such as color and size, and enhanced existing features, such as larger numerals of higher contrast, would also benefit those with normal vision by making denomination more rapid and convenient for all.

REFERENCES

Abbott, G. 1994. Presentation to the Committee on Currency Features Usable by the Visually Impaired. March 30, 1994.

Benson, V., and M.A. Marano. 1994. Current estimates from the National Health Interview Survey. National Center for Health Statistics, January 1994. Vital and Health Statistics Series 10(189):95.

Cholewiak, R. 1994. Presentation to the Committee on Currency Features Usable by the Visually Impaired. March 30, 1994.

Genensky, S. 1978. Data concerning the partially sighted and functionally blind. Journal of Visual Impairment and Blindness 72(5):177–180.

Genensky, S. 1994. Personal communication to the Committee on Currency Features Usable by the Visually Impaired. March 30, 1994.

Jewish Guild for the Blind, The. 1992. Photos taken from visual impairment poster. New York: The Jewish Guild for the Blind.

Laming, D. R. J. 1986. Sensory Analysis. San Diego, California: Academic Press.

Legge, G.E. 1991. Glenn A. Fry Award Lecture 1990: Three perspectives on low-vision reading. Optometry and Vision Science 68:763–769.

Legge, G.E. 1993. The role of contrast in reading: Normal and low vision. Pp. 269–287 in Contrast Sensitivity, R.M. Shipley and D.M.-K. Lam, eds. Cambridge, Massachusetts: Massachusetts Institute of Technology Press.

Legge, G.E. 1994. Presentation to the Committee on Currency Features Usable by the Visually Impaired. February 23, 1994.

Legge, G.E., G.S. Rubin, and A. Luebker. 1987. Psychophysics of reading. V. The role of contrast in normal vision. Vision Research 27:1165–1171.

Maurer, M. 1994. Presentation to the Committee on Currency Features Usable by the Visually Impaired. March 29, 1994.

Miller G. 1956. The magical number seven plus or minus two: Some limits on our capacity for processing information. Psychological Review 63(2):81–97.

National Advisory Eye Council. 1993. Vision Research—A National Plan: 1994–1998. National Institutes of Health Publication No. 93-3186.

NRC (National Research Council). 1994. Measurement of Visual Field and Visual Acuity for Disability Determination. National Research Council Committee on Vision, NRC. Washington, D.C.: National Academy Press.

Nelson, K. A., and E. Dimitrova. 1993. Severe visual impairment in the United States and in each state, 1990. Journal Visual Impairment and Blindness 87(3):80–85.

Pitts, D. G. 1982. The effects of aging on selected visual functions: Dark adaptation, visual acuity, stereopsis, and brightness contrast. Pp. 131–159 in Aging and Human Visual Function, R. Sekuler, D. Kline, and K. Dismukes, eds. New York: Alan R. Liss, Inc.

RPFFB (RP Foundation Fighting Blindness). 1994. Information about Usher Syndrome. Baltimore, Maryland: National Retinitis Pigmentosa Foundation, Inc., RP Foundation Fighting Blindness.

RSVFP (Randolph-Sheppard Vending Facility Program). 1993. Annual Report, Fiscal Year 1992. Washington, D.C.: Office of Special Education and Rehabilitative Services, U.S. Department of Education.

Rubin, G.S., and G.E. Legge. 1989. Psychophysics of reading. VI. The role of contrast in low vision. Vision Research 29:79–91.

Schreier, E. 1994. Presentation to the Committee on Currency Features Usable by the Visually Impaired. March 30, 1994.

Tielsch, J.M., A. Sommer, K. Witt, J. Katz, and R.M. Royall. 1990. Blindness and visual impairment in an American urban population: The Baltimore eye survey. Archives of Ophthalmology 108:286–290.

World Health Organization. 1966. Blindness Information Collected from Various Sources. Epidemiology and Vital Statistics Report 19:427–511.

3

ASSESSMENT METHODOLOGY FOR FEATURES FOR VISUALLY IMPAIRED PEOPLE

REQUIREMENTS

Introducing banknote features to allow people who are visually disabled to recognize, denominate, and authenticate U.S. banknotes requires identification of the most effective feature or combinations of features. In general, the feature(s) should be (1) easy to use and reliable; (2) long-wearing, maintaining readability over the life of the banknote; (3) benign, not significantly degrading banknote durability; (4) cost-effective for the BEP to implement; (5) difficult to simulate; and (6) relatively inexpensive for the population to use.

From the large list of possible features assembled by the committee, it is necessary to assess individual features and combinations of features to identify an optimum set that addresses all of these issues. One aspect of evaluating the proposed features is the development of operational meanings for the terms "recognize,""denominate," and "authenticate" and the determination of how well each feature performs these individual tasks. Figure 3-1 indicates a logical sequence that a person may follow when handed a banknote. First, there is the recognition that the piece of paper is represented by the giver to be a banknote; then, the value of the banknote is determined; finally, the banknote is verified as authentic. In this sequence, the definition of "authentication" encompasses the definitions of the other two; that is, if a banknote is verified as authentic, it is both determined to be a genuine U.S. banknote (as opposed to another document or counterfeit), and its value is known. Since individual features have varying strengths in identifying either the legitimacy of the banknote or its denomination, these two elements of authentication will be addressed separately. In this report, the term "authenticate" will be restricted to mean to verify a banknote as a genuine U.S. banknote; the term "denominate" will be used to mean to determine the value of the banknote. Lastly, the term "recognize" will be used to mean to differentiate the banknote from other pieces of paper of similar size, for example, store receipts. While it is the primary goal of this committee to recommend features that will help visually disabled people to recognize and denominate banknotes, the committee also evaluated features that will also help them authenticate banknotes.

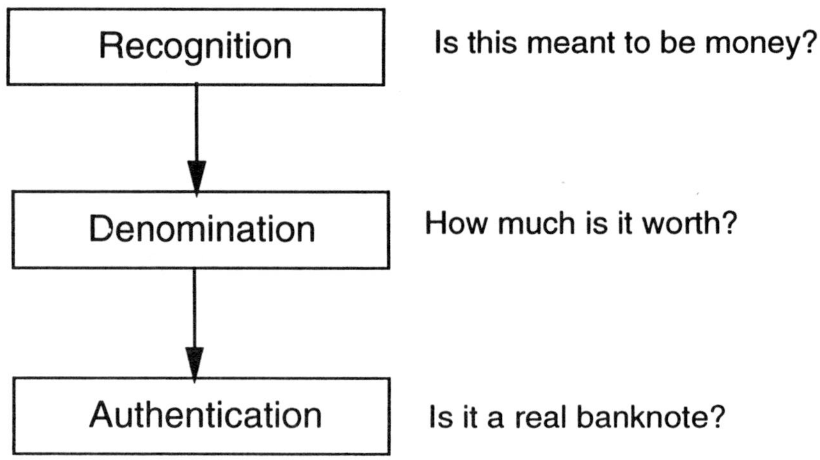

Figure 3-1 Logical sequence of banknote verification: recognition-denomination-authentication.

THE IDEAL FEATURE

It is instructive to describe the "ideal" feature for recognizing; denominating; and, if possible, authenticating banknotes as a model to compare with "real" features. The committee gained some insight by summarizing the attributes of an ideal counterfeit-deterrent feature as they were described in previous reports (NRC, 1993; Church and Littman, 1992). These attributes are as follows:

- difficult to duplicate;
- difficult to simulate;
- easily recognized by the general public;
- durable (i.e., the feature is useful even after considerable wear);
- easy to produce at low cost;
- can cocirculate with current banknotes;
- acceptable to the public (aesthetically pleasing);
- machine readable; and
- nontoxic and nonhazardous.

While the previous NRC study concentrated on optical or visible features to deter counterfeiting (NRC, 1993), many of these attributes are also desirable in a feature to be used by visually disabled people to recognize and denominate U.S. banknotes. An ideal feature for visually disabled people would also

- reliably indicate the denomination of the banknote;
- reliably indicate the orientation of the banknote;
- address the needs of the whole population, from blind people to the normally sighted; and
- be easy to use (i.e., not require a device or extended handling).

No feature that the committee evaluated was considered ideal by these criteria, so the committee took the approach of identifying the ability of a given feature or combination of features to satisfy individual criteria, then weighing the relative importance of the evaluation criteria to come up with an optimized set of recommendations. The committee also carried out a similar analysis for devices for denominating banknotes. The discussion of this analysis is found in Chapter 4.

EVALUATION STRATEGY

The list of features to evaluate was very long, and each feature had several variations. In the present study to evaluate and compare a disparate group of possible features, the committee took a similar approach to that taken in the consideration of counterfeit-deterrent currency features. That is, the committee identified a set of requirements that may be stated initially in vague or general terms, converted the requirements into indicators or criteria; weighted the criteria in terms of their relative importance; and scored or ranked the alternatives with reference to the criteria.

In addition to the purely "technical" evaluation described above, the committee considered the target populations for the individual features. A feature that might be of considerable assistance to those with normal or low vision might not benefit blind people at all. Since there may be a relatively large population that would benefit from the feature, the committee chose to recommend that feature despite the fact that it would not be universally useful. The committee also considered features that may be of principal benefit to people who are blind, which might not be particularly useful to those with some vision. The committee attempted to ensure that their list of recommended features provided overlapping coverage, so that each of the target groups would gain significant benefits from the redesigned banknotes if those recommended features were included.

EVALUATION FRAMEWORK

The committee developed four categories of evaluation criteria: population, function, technical success, and implementation success. Each of these four categories was further subdivided into the criteria against which all proposed features were graded. Figure 3-2 shows the specific criteria in the general categories, and tables 3-1 through 3-4 list the criteria in each group with a short explanation of what is considered "success" for each criterion.

The first two general categories are relatively self-explanatory—who will use this feature (population category), and what information about the banknote will the person get using this feature (function category). The third category, technical success criteria, expresses the committee's impression of the ability of the feature to succeed based on technical aspects such as the ease of use, resistance to false positives, etc. The final category, implementation success criteria, takes into account the way that a particular feature would be implemented by the BEP and its impact on circulation.

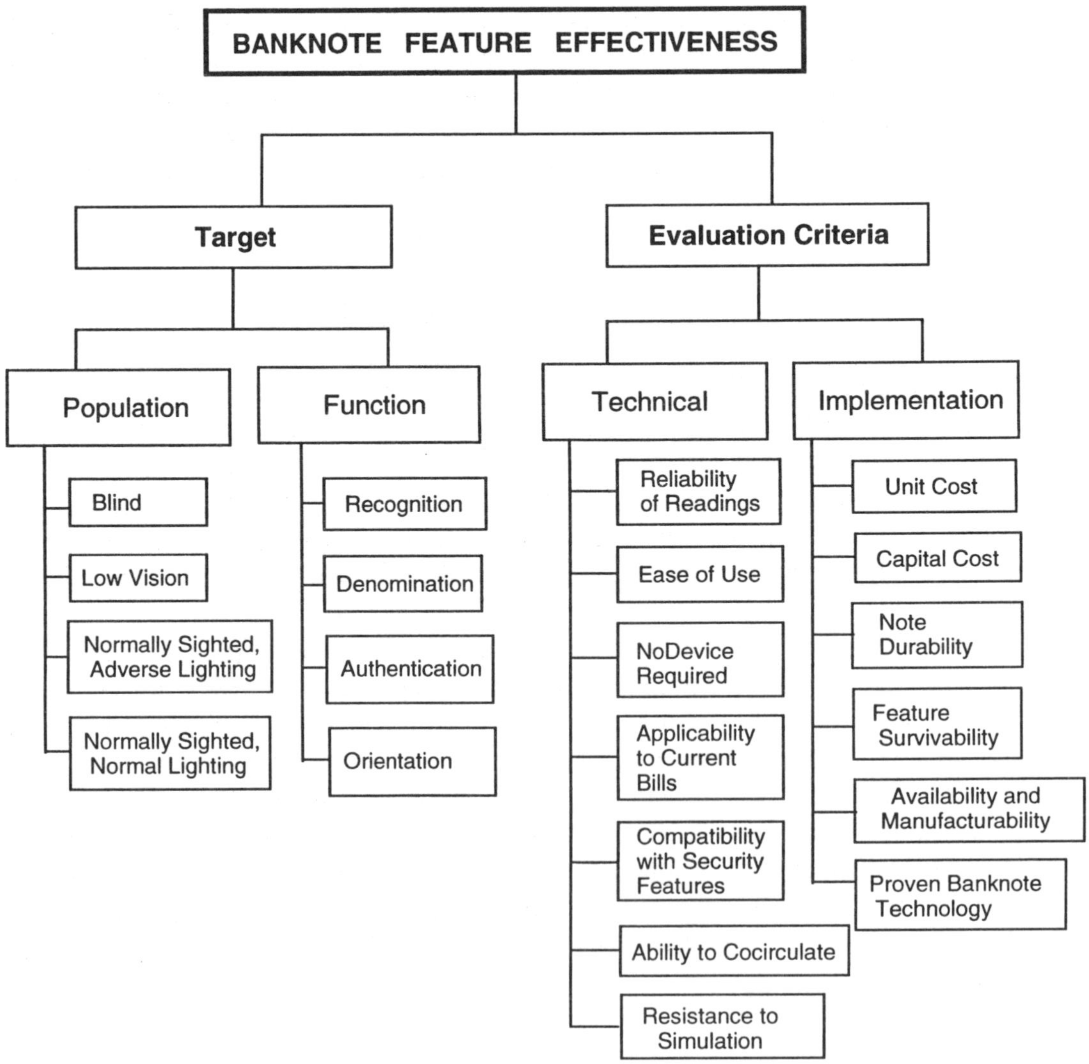

Figure 3-2 Evaluation criteria used to determine the effectiveness of proposed currency features.

For example, punching holes in banknotes, with the number of holes indicating denomination, would be assessed as a general concept in the technical success probability category, with some positive and some negative attributes. In the implementation success criteria category, the shape of the hole (for example, star-shaped, round, or oval) would need to be known for evaluation against criteria such as feature survivability or note durability. The committee's assumption about how a particular feature would be implemented was noted when the feature was evaluated. The various ways a feature could be implemented are discussed in chapters 4 and 6.

The committee gave more weight to certain criteria in each category. In the first category, features that would be useful to people who are blind and those with low vision were given more weight. In the function category, the major weight was placed on denomination, as opposed to

Table 3-1 Population Category

Category	Description of a Successful Feature
Blind	Blind people can use the feature
Low Vision	People with low vision can use the feature
Normally Sighted, Adverse Lighting	Normally sighted people can use the feature in low light
Normally Sighted, Normal Lighting	Normally sighted people can use the feature in normal light

Table 3-2 Function Category

Category	Description of a Successful Feature
Recognition	Feature can be used to differentiate banknotes from other similar-sized paper
Denomination	Feature can be used to determine the value of the banknote
Authentication	Feature can be used to determine if the note is a genuine U.S. banknote
Orientation	Feature can be used to orient banknotes for use in vending and other machines

authentication, recognition, or orientation. Authentication (in the committee's strict definition) is not thought to be more of a problem for visually disabled people than for the rest of the population, but features that could be used for authentication as well as denomination were rated more highly than features that were only useful for denomination. Orientation of banknotes is necessary for many vending machines and for bank deposits (mostly from businesses, where large amounts of cash are regularly brought into the bank), so it is included as a desirable attribute but not an essential one.

In the final two categories, technical success risk and implementation success risk, the criteria were not strictly ranked but were thought of as "high" weight or "low" weight. In the category for technical success criteria, the criteria considered to be most important were

- reliability of readings;
- ease of use;
- compatibility with security features;
- no requirement for a device other than a person's senses; and
- resistance to simulation.

Table 3-3 Technical Success Criteria

Category	Description of a Successful Feature
Reliability of Readings	Readings do not give "false positives," (i.e., they do not indicate that a note is a denomination other than its true value) or "false negatives" (reject valid banknotes)
Ease of Use	Feature is easy to use, especially in a situation where there is little time to examine money
No Requirement for Device	A person's senses can be used to evaluate the banknote, with no requirement for any device or machine
Applicability to Current Banknotes	Feature could be applied to currency presently in circulation or production without a redesign
Compatible with Security Features	Feature is compatible with security features scheduled for implementation in the new currency design or recommended in the previous report (NRC, 1993)
Ability to Cocirculate	Notes can cocirculate with present notes without confusion, misidentification or compromise of automated money-handling machines
Resistance to Simulation	Feature cannot be easily simulated or corrupted to indicate another denomination

Table 3-4 Implementation Success Criteria

Category	Description of a Successful Feature
Unit Cost	Unit cost for note production (cost per note) is low
Capital Cost	Capital cost to BEP and Federal Reserve is low
Durability of Banknote	The feature will not significantly reduce durability below that of present banknotes
Survivability of Feature	Feature will serve its intended use after wear and tear of handling and circulation
Availability and Manufacturability	Technology to manufacture banknotes with the feature is available now
Proven Banknote Technology	Feature has been used before on banknotes in other countries

In the category for implementation success criteria, the most important criteria were

- survivability of the feature;
- durability of the banknote;
- capital cost; and
- availability and manufacturability.

Capital costs were considered too high at the point where a complete line of additional printing equipment would be required. A new line of equipment may also have an impact on unit costs. Changes to existing operating equipment or modifications to parts of the equipment were considered to be acceptable in terms of capital and unit costs.

The list of proposed features was organized generally into groups, including substrate based, edge modification, tactile marking, visual marking, and other. The proposed features were evaluated against the criteria described in these tables, using a "yes," "no," or "maybe" to indicate whether the feature met each criterion for success, whether it did not meet the criterion, or whether the committee was not able to evaluate whether the proposed feature met the criterion. For the cost criterion, the full costs of implementation, including costs beyond those incurred by the BEP, were considered to be outside the scope of the present work. The ideal feature for use by visually disabled people would have been rated "yes" in all categories.

If a feature was evaluated a *no* or a *maybe* for a certain criterion, the committee discussed whether the shortcoming of that feature was a fundamental limitation of the feature or whether the technology required for the feature to be useful and realizable could benefit from further development work. Features that fit into the latter category were noted as candidates for future research (see Chapter 5). Compatibility with security features may be highly important for the near term. Incompatibility with security features proposed for implementation in the long term is not as serious a negative factor, since research and development work to be done for the security feature may determine a way to improve compatibility.

Further criteria were needed for any feature that required the use of a device for denominating banknotes. Some features, while not accessible to a person's unaided senses, may make it easier to design a simple and convenient device to denominate banknotes. This type of device could have widespread use in the vending community and may be necessary for those who cannot use other features implemented. Features in this category will be evaluated in Chapter 4, along with features that allow for unaided banknote denomination. The types of devices that the committee envisions will be developed are also discussed in Chapter 4. An additional set of criteria was developed for the evaluation of the devices themselves.

When considering the use of devices, the committee identified various criteria that would contribute to successful implementation of a device. In addition, the committee outlined various performance-related criteria that need to be fulfilled when a device is operated in a realistic environment.

The criteria for evaluating devices were the following (in no specific order):

- ability to recognize and denominate;
- highly accurate;
- private;

- small/portable;
- low maintenance;
- inexpensive/good value;
- rapid response;
- low power consumption; and
- long lived.

Future development of denomination devices might emphasize the ability to authenticate banknotes as well as to denominate them. The term "inexpensive" is coupled with "good value" to indicate that the amount that a person would be willing to pay for a device is directly related to how useful that device would be. That is, a small, easily used device might be a good value at a higher price than a larger, slower device. If a device receives a satisfactory rating for all of the above criteria, then its operational characteristics for performance should include:

- a low-false-reject rate;
- independence of note orientation;
- an acceptable operating temperature/humidity range; and
- easy use by untrained/unskilled individuals.

These criteria are shown in Figure 3-3 as a diagram, which is similar to that drawn up for feature criteria in Figure 3-2.

The form of a device's output characteristics should take into account potential international usage and could be audible (multilingual), tactile, or visual.

When discussing many of the above points the committee formed the opinion that the technology could be helpful to people with normal vision using point-of-sale devices, cash accepting machines and automated cash registers, etc. This wider use may well increase the respective market for the units, bringing the prices down and driving the performance upwards.

Finally, a list of recommended features was drawn up, with notations as to what questions still need to be answered before implementation. Features were grouped by the way in which a user would get information about the banknote, whether they are visual/tactile (information from both sight and touch), visual only (information from sight), tactile only (information from touch), or machine-readable (information from a device that "reads" the feature and interprets the banknote information for the user).

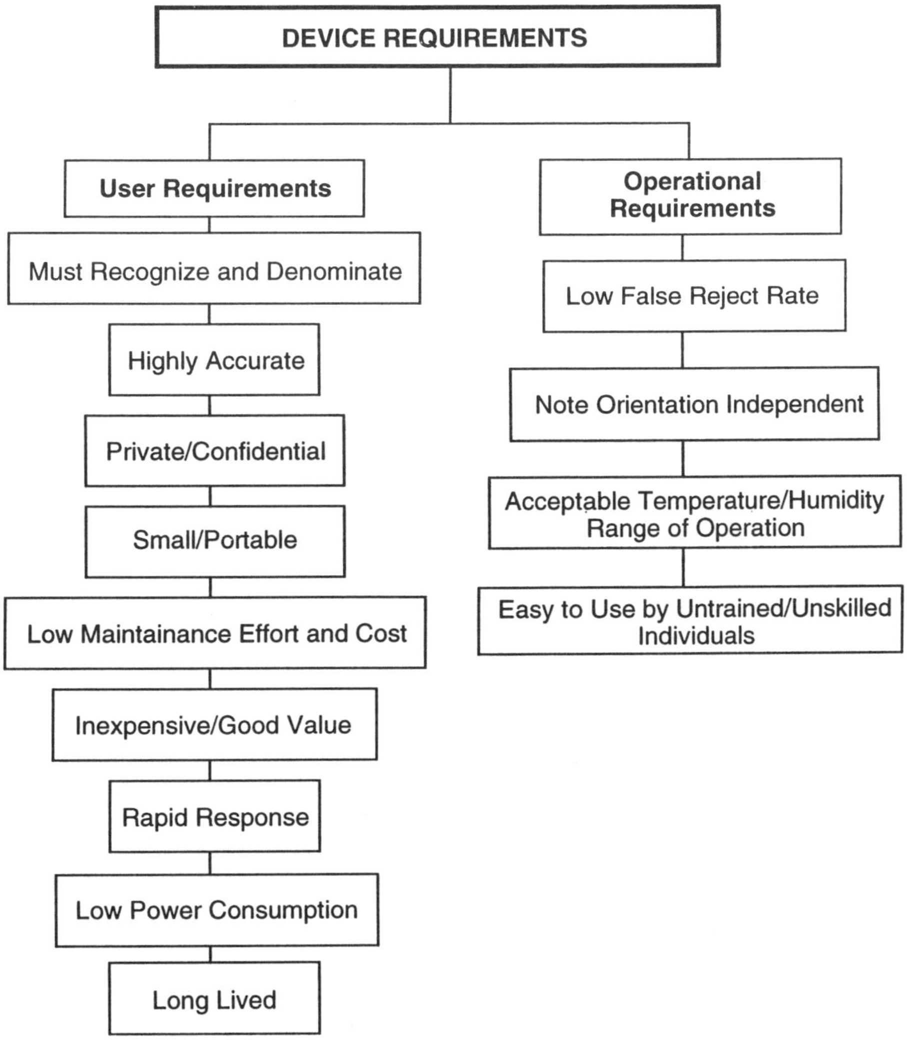

Figure 3-3 Evaluation criteria for banknote denomination/authentication devices.

REFERENCES

Church, S., and D. Littman. 1992. Presentation by Sara Church, Bureau of Engraving and Printing, and Dan Littman, Federal Reserve System, to the Committee on Next-Generation Currency Design. October 21, 1992.

NRC (National Research Council). 1993. Counterfeit Deterrent Features for the Next-Generation Currency Design. NMAB-472. National Materials Advisory Board, NRC. Washington, D.C.: National Academy Press.

4

DESCRIPTION AND ASSESSMENT OF FEATURES

The importance of assisting visually disabled people was not addressed at the time the current U.S. banknotes were first issued in 1929, and the notes were manufactured using then-available technology. In a world of mainly monochromatic commercial print, the 1929 designs with their characteristic green backs were easily recognizable.

As the twentieth century comes to an end, everyone is aware of visual and tactile presentations that distinguish and sell items in daily life. Television and supermarkets are models on how to mix a multitude of similar products and yet achieve separation by techniques of brand identification. The awareness that different groupings of the population can be specifically addressed is now well understood. It is against this background that the committee has looked at features that could be incorporated into the U.S. banknotes to aid visually disabled people to recognize the presence of a banknote, identifying its denomination and, if possible, providing secure authentication.

A list of such features was drawn up from a variety of sources. The features were ones used or recommended by foreign currency issuers (see Appendix D), discussed in previous studies, suggested by participants in the workshop held by the committee, and identified by committee members. Some features on the original list were currently considered too impractical for complete evaluation. These features are listed in Appendix E. To make the evaluation easier to comprehend, the committee decided that the best method for grouping the features was to address how information would be obtained by the user. By combining the target population with the methods of identification, the following four major groupings were identified: visual/tactile features, visual-only features, tactile-only features, and machine-readable features. Figures 4-1 and 4-2 show examples of some of the various features that the committee considered; the features illustrated in these figures will be discussed in their appropriate chapter section.

VISUAL/TACTILE FEATURES

Features in this category give both visual and tactile clues to the denomination and would be usable by both blind and sighted people. These include features that may be incorporated into the substrate during manufacture, for example, changes in the physical dimensions of the note or features that involve modification of the substrate after manufacture, such as modification of the corners or edges or the addition of holes.

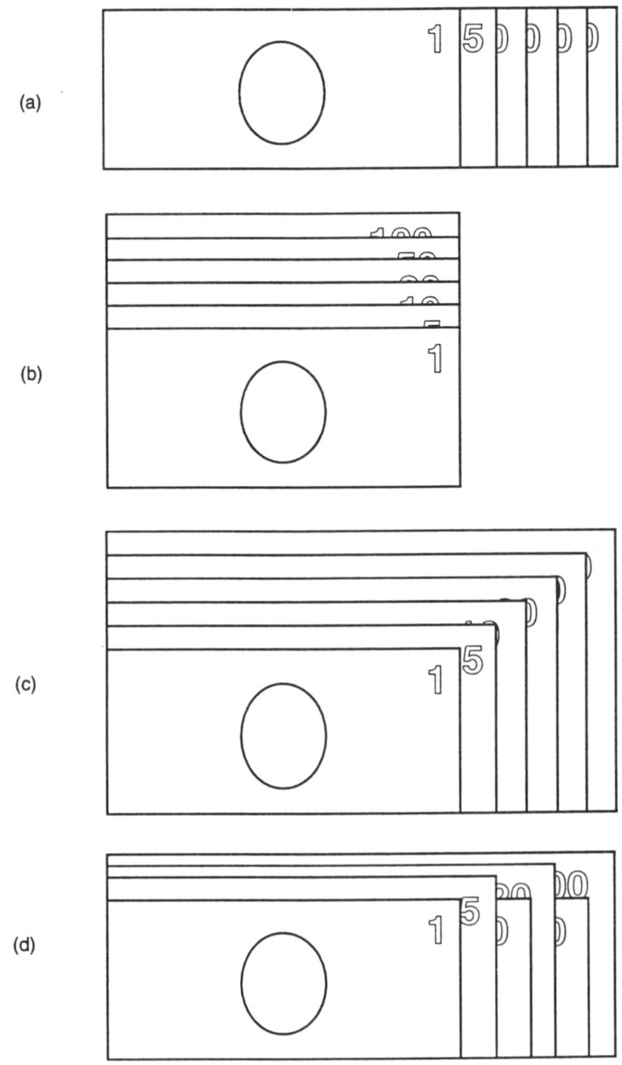

Figure 4-1 Illustrations of various ways to use size to indicate banknote denomination: (a) length only; (b) height only; (c) both length and height; (d) hybrid use of length and height.

Size

Conceptually, the simplest visual/tactile approach is to have different-sized notes, where the size indicates the denomination (see Figure 4-1). This is an established practice in over 120 countries in the world (see table in Appendix D). The length, height, or both dimensions of the note can be changed depending on denomination. The usual practice is to have the higher denominations of a larger size, so that the crime of "raising" the value cannot be achieved.

Figure 4-1 illustrates the types of dimensional changes possible. Figures 4-1a and 4-1b show single-dimension variations of length and height, respectively. Figure 4-1c shows an increase in both length and height for each increase in denomination. A combination of length changes with alternating changes in height is shown as a "hybrid model" in Figure 4-1d.

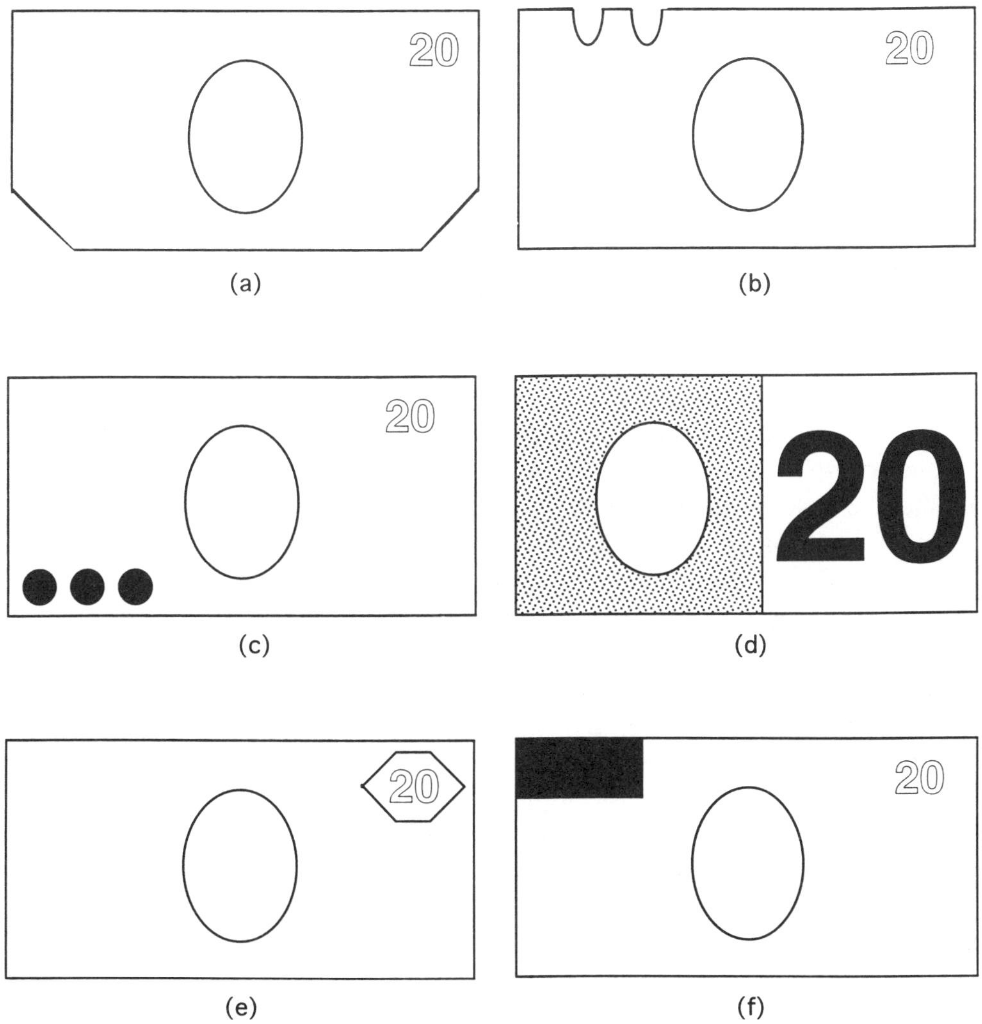

Figure 4-2 Illustrations of various features evaluated: (a) corner cuts; (b) edge notches; (c) holes; (d) large numerals, uncluttered background; (e) distinctive shapes; (f) coarse patterns. (Features in (a) and (b) have been exaggerated for illustration purposes.)

In countries where the currency is size-denominated, organizations representing and supporting blind people, such as the Royal National Institute of the Blind and the European Blind Union, recommend continuation of this practice (EBU, 1994; Farber, 1994; King, 1994; Jarvis, 1994). The use of this feature in U.S. banknotes has been an ongoing recommendation by those who are familiar with the use of different-sized banknotes and is considered to be extremely useful once an individual is trained to use it. Participants in the committee's workshop also recommended the use of size-denominated banknotes, based on their experiences in traveling and living in other countries and in handling coins and other size-differentiated objects (Hill, 1994; Miller, 1994; Wallach, 1994; Abbott, 1994).

Sizing banknotes by denomination does not provide any clue to the orientation of the bill other than identification of length versus height. To give orientation information, an additional feature would be necessary. Such a feature would not need to give information about a bill's denomination.

The committee found no technical literature evaluating the effectiveness of denomination differentiation by size other than a mention in a paper evaluating the effectiveness of the tactile marks used on Dutch currency (Koeze, 1990). In that paper, one subject who identified all denominations correctly 100 percent of the time used banknote size, although distinctive tactile markings were available. The BEP report (1983) indicates that there was research done by the Central Bank of Switzerland that indicated the usefulness of size-denominated banknotes for blind people. Generally, there is little published literature directly related to banknote features due to the confidentiality with which currency design, handling, and production are treated.

To the committee's knowledge, careful psychophysical measurements have not been reported on size discrimination and identification in a context directly applicable to currency bills. Tactile judgments of the size of bills involve active exploration with the hands and fingers. This type of "active touch" makes use of sensory inputs from both touch receptors on the skin (cutaneous sense) and positional receptors in the muscles and joints of the hands and fingers (kinesthetic sense). Basic psychophysical studies have tended to isolate each of these two components of tactile perception for separate study. For example, Durlach et al. (1989) performed a detailed study of tactile length discrimination and identification using judgments of distance between the thumb and forefinger (the kinesthetic sense). For a length of 80 mm, the Weber fraction was 3 percent (2.4 mm), but the Weber fraction increased slightly for shorter lengths. The Weber fraction of 3 percent was consistent with earlier measurements of length discrimination and represents the committee's best available estimate of a lower bound of appropriate length differences for banknote design. In the same study, Durlach et al. also confirmed the point made in Chapter 2 regarding absolute judgment; even if length differences exceed the discrimination threshold, errors of absolute judgment occur when the number of alternatives exceeds about four to seven.

Based on the limited technical data and the strong recommendations for this feature from blind communities in Europe, some very preliminary experiments were carried out by two members of the committee to examine these aspects (Legge, 1994; Brabyn, 1994). Legge concentrated on size variation in length only. Six "banknotes" with 6 mm differences between "denominations" (mean length of 156 mm), could be identified with 50 percent accuracy. When the step size was increased to 12 mm, identification improved to 75 percent accurate. Brabyn showed that using four sizes of notes that varied in size in two dimensions—length by 7 mm and height by 5 mm—a 90 percent success rate for identification could be achieved in a short learning time (about one-half hour). The coding of both length and height can be thought of as a special case of the addition of a secondary cue to ease identification, which is described in the discussion of discrimination versus absolute judgment in Chapter 2. More work is needed to identify the optimum sizes, but this needs to involve the BEP to ensure that the cost efficiencies of different sizes, including plate layout considerations, are also taken into account.

To determine the optimum set of sizes for six denominations, the approaches used by the many countries that include this denomination cue in their currency should be evaluated. In addition, the threshold differences in dimension required between two adjacent denominations need to be examined to add a technical basis for the choice of sizes. For steps to safely exceed the Weber fraction for length, they will probably need to be at least 3 percent of the base length.

The European Blind Union recommends a minimum difference of 5 mm between denominations (EBU, 1994). Such differences could lead to extra-large notes. Most countries use a second cue to improve performance. This can often take the form of a template that is provided at the launch of the new notes design to provide improved discrimination. Alternatively, the notes can vary in two dimensions; this is the norm and is also recommended by the European Blind Union (EBU, 1994). With this option, the examiner has two edges to relate judgment against. Often the hand replaces the template as a known guide, using, for example, the distance from the thumb joint up the first finger.

In the 1983 BEP report, a table contains the dimensions of currencies issued by 38 countries (BEP, 1983).[1] From the information listed in the BEP table, 36 countries varied both dimensions of the banknote, and the Netherlands and Israel varied banknote length only. Most of the dimensional changes are not linear through the series of banknote denominations; that is, the step size from one denomination to the next larger denomination is not constant through the entire denomination sequence. Step sizes in both length and width generally fell between 4 mm and 16 mm, with some as small as 1 mm or as large as 28 mm. According to the table, the Netherlands and Israel increased banknote length by 6 mm and 7 mm per step, respectively. Design and plate layout considerations generally dictate the choice of step sizes between successive denominations.

There have been general comments that variations in sizes will affect the use of ATMs (automatic teller machines) and other cash-handling machines. Although some alterations would be necessary, the committee was made aware that these machines are also used in Europe where banknote sizes vary with denomination. Recently both England and Germany have issued new series of banknotes that have different sizes than the previous notes. Despite a complicated multiplicity of sizes, the providers of ATM services were able to keep the machines working. U.S.-manufactured ATMs are used throughout the world in countries with size-denominated banknotes.

A previous report (BEP, 1983) indicated that size changes were the most effective way to denominate banknotes for the visually disabled but that such changes would be costly. At the time that report was issued, there was no currency redesign anticipated, and their cost estimates included the full costs of redesigning the currency. The committee recommends that the calculation be revisited, taking into account the fact that a currency redesign is underway and based on present banknote manufacturing equipment employed and the current distribution of denominational production. For example, over 40 percent of production consists of $1 bills (Church, 1994). These would become the smallest notes under a varying size policy. Smaller notes would mean that more notes could be produced on each sheet, thus leading to savings in paper, ink, and production time. Against this, some capital equipment would require replacement, and methods of handling the finished product by BEP and the Federal Reserve banks would need changes. In addition to the BEP and Federal Reserve bank costs, there would be conversion costs for vending and other cash-handling machines outside the BEP and Federal Reserve banks, as well as other "downstream" costs to merchants and individuals.

---

[1] Banknote designs change frequently around the world, so the numbers in the BEP report are not current. A summary is presented as an indication of the types of dimensional variations used.

Although there is a substantial infrastructure in the United States that relies on single-sized banknotes, the committee believes that the needs of the visually impaired would be well-served by making the banknotes size-denominated. Because of the strong recommendations from members of the target communities who have experience using this feature and because of the amount of experience worldwide in the manufacture and use of this technology, the committee recommends that the BEP work to implement size-denominated banknotes to ease use of U.S. currency by all.

Edge Modification

Another variation of substrate dimension changes is to notch, cut corners, or modify edges of the note, as depicted in figures 4-2a and 4-2b. Clipping corners has been considered by other countries but is not currently in use. Similar to the case of dimensional changes above, lower denomination bills would have more corners cut. For example, the $100 bill could have no corners cut off; the $50 bill, one corner (perhaps, the lower left); the $20 bill, two corners (the lower left and right); the $10 bill, a different two corners (the lower left and upper left); the $5 bill, three corners (lower left and right and upper left); and the $1 note could have all four corners cut. In this scheme, the cut corner approach would provide an orientation cue, except in the case of the one or one hundred dollar notes.

In the committee's opinion, cutting the corners of the note would not be expected to increase the possibility of failure by delamination of the paper layers and, in fact, may lessen this tendency. There would be capital cost associated with this feature, since means to cut the corners or make notches would be required. Because folded corners could be confused with cut corners by both people and machines, this approach is not considered suitable as a primary denomination cue.

Edge modifications to the note could be a notch with square or rounded corners cut into the banknote edge (see Figure 4-2b). A sharp notch may have a tendency to enhance delamination or tearing, whereas a more gradual pattern should not. Such edge patterns, in addition to helping with denomination, could also provide information on the orientation of the note for a blind person and help to stack notes of the same denomination in piles. Denominating the notes could be accomplished using a pattern on one edge only or on multiple edges.

The patterned edges could be thought of as aids much like the edges of coins. For example, edge patterns could help distinguish between nearest neighbor denominations or could complement note size features (mentioned above) for sizes that are close. As will be discussed later, corner clipping and edge modifications could both be used in combination with size changes. For instance, clipping the corner of alternate denominations would improve accuracy in denomination and aid in orientation of the bill.

As in the case of cut corners, there will be some capital cost associated with the edge modification feature. For cut corners or other edge modifications, the potential for enhanced degradation of the note, while believed by the committee to be small, must be evaluated. Because the concerns in handling and degradation with wear, the modification of banknote edges does not appear to the committee to be a reasonable approach at this time.

Holes

Holes punched or drilled into the note offer another opportunity for both orientation and denomination. Holes should be simple and inexpensive to implement, and the denomination information could be carried by the location of the holes, the number of holes (see Figure 4-2c), or both. In addition, this approach would provide definite orientation information if the "active" quadrant was always the same. For example, if the holes were confined to the lower left quadrant of the front of the note for all denominations, it would be easy to orient the bill properly. The idea of holes was presented to the committee (Oschwald and Hendricks, 1994) and has received limited field testing with encouraging results. During these experiments, a template with raised bumps that would be felt through the holes was used to enable reliable detection. There is some debate as to the efficiency of detecting holes by feel alone. The committee was informed that depressed areas are more difficult to detect from a background than raised areas, so that holes significantly larger than braille dots would be required for accurate identification. Holes in the interior of the banknote could also be "read" by folding the note along the line of the holes and feeling the notches along the folded edge. This method combines the benefits of an edge modification, where the notches are easily distinguished, with the improved robustness of having the holes in the banknote interior, where they are less likely to start tears or delamination problems or to jam the transport mechanisms of currency-handling machines. However, continued folding along the same line will cause banknote degradation.

Production implementation would require assessment, since a drilling apparatus will be necessary. Circular holes are straightforward to drill compared with shaped holes. The cost of drilling should also be cheaper than edge modifications or corner cutting. However, the impact of increasing the number of processing steps and wastage of material will need to be assessed together with durability. The committee believes that circular holes would be more durable than shaped holes. It also felt that larger holes, which would be more easily located and identified, would be more vulnerable to damage than small holes, thus a balance of perception requirements versus durability for hole size would need investigating. One drawback to the scheme of holes is that punching a hole in a document is often carried out in commercial transactions to denote that an item has no monetary worth.

Because the concept of using hole location or number of holes to indicate banknote denomination is very simple and would be easy to use, the committee believes that it would be worthwhile for the BEP to assess such issues as the impact of holes on banknote durability and the psychological matters regarding issuing and using banknotes containing holes.

VISUAL-ONLY FEATURES

Visual-only features would benefit everyone except people who are blind. These types of features include large numerals on a nonprinted background (to obtain high contrast), printed geometrical shapes unique to the denomination of the note, coarse printed patterns that would correspond to note value, and different colors for different note values. None of these features would provide for authentication of the note.

Numerals

The use of large, high-contrast numerals on a simple, uniform background can provide an effective means to enable visually disabled people to more easily denominate banknotes. "Large" here refers to numerals greater than 40 percent of the full height of the current note (see Figure 4-2d). This size would be well within the limit of people with acuity of 20/160 or better for viewing bills at a distance of one meter, which is roughly the distance from the eye to the checkout counter of a grocery store, enabling easy and rapid identification. (See the discussion in Chapter 2 dealing with acuity levels and currency identification.) If the numeral were 60 percent of the current note height, it would serve people with acuity as low as 20/240 in the same situation. Moreover, the large, easy-to-read numerals would be recognizable by people with extremely low acuities (less than 20/1000) if bills were held at a normal reading distance of 40 cm (16 inches). Numerals of this size would be substantially larger than those on current U.S. banknotes. Large numerals are not needed on all four corners, but it would be preferable that one large numeral be included on each side of the banknote. However, a large numeral on one side only would provide an additional orientation cue.

Large numerals may offer a location for additional anticounterfeiting features, such as finely detailed numeral-edge engraving. The overall high contrast with the background must be maintained, however. Large numerals may also distract from finely engraved security features, such as the portrait work, so care must be taken to integrate the numerals into the design in such a way that distraction is minimized.

Along with the larger numerals must be a plain, uncluttered background to provide high contrast for easy readability. Large numerals on a plain background are common in foreign currency and were recommended by organizations supporting visually disabled people (EBU, 1994; Farber, 1994; Bennett, 1994). Current U.S. notes do not, in general, offer much contrast. Photometric measurements performed by a committee member show that contrast ranges from 30 percent (worn) to 60 percent (new; Legge, 1994). A National Research Council committee recommended in 1980 a minimum contrast of 85 percent for symbols used in acuity testing (NRC, 1980); this should be used as a starting point for design of a high contrast numeral. The size of the clear background needed relative to the size of the numeral is uncertain at this point and would likely require additional study. A reasonable starting assumption, however, is that the surrounding clear field should be at least the width of the lines forming the character. The numeral could be either white on a black background or black on a white background. People with light scatter in the ocular media (e.g., cataract) often see better with white characters on a dark background, so an argument can be made for the merits of white on black. However, dark numerals on a light background, as can be found on the new Canadian $20 note, may stand out as a "target" against a light background better than a light numeral on a dark background.

Large, high-contrast numerals are simple to implement; the only concern is where to place large numerals in the crowded design. The committee believes that a large portion of the visually disabled would be served by the implementation of this feature.

Color

Color can serve as a denomination aid if each note value is assigned a different predominant color. For example, a $5 bill could be predominantly blue. A person with low vision who could not make out the numerals (large or otherwise) may be able to discern color differences to determine the denomination. The use of color could also be a convenient aid for the normally sighted. This feature would require learning the colors associated with a given note value.

It is customary in currency design for each denomination to have a single, predominant color. That color is usually on both sides of the banknote, so that notes can be distinguished by viewing either banknote face. However, if a denominating color is only on one side of the note, the color feature could also assist in front to back orientation. Having the denominating color on the front of the banknote is preferable, since people tend to orient banknotes with the front face toward the user. If policy is to require the fronts of the banknotes to be printed in black, then a second choice would be to apply a distinctive predominant color to the banknote backs. Although an argument can be made that a complicated color design with a mix of colors on one face may be a counterfeit deterrent, it is not considered desirable from a denomination standpoint.

The color observed by the eye is dependent on the spectral content of the illumination source, so colors selected for banknotes would have to remain distinct under varied lighting conditions. For example, certain blues and greens can be hard to distinguish from each other in low light or by people with low vision; banknotes should not be designed to rely on discrimination between such colors. There is enough information in the area of color research to allow experts in the field to identify six colors that could distinguish the six denominations with little research or development needed (Arditi, 1994). The committee is aware that other aesthetic and design considerations may place some restrictions on the choice of a set of colors. In addition, color choices should be made that will not result in confusion for the 10 percent of the population (mostly male) with inherited color deficits.

Existing printing technology at the BEP offers two ways to apply color to the banknote: intaglio printing and letter press printing. (Lithographic printing is used in other countries to apply color to banknotes, but it is not used at the BEP.) For printing an entire face in one color, the intaglio press is used. The intaglio equipment at the BEP is capable of printing three separate colors in each print run. As a banknote is printed, the press uses either green ink (for the banknote back) or black ink (for the front of the banknote). Between denomination runs, the intaglio press is cleaned, and the plates are changed to the appropriate denomination plates. At the same time as the operator cleans the machine and changes the plates, the ink can be changed with little additional work. Since so many other countries use different-colored intaglio inks, there is little limitation to the number of color choices available off-the-shelf. The availability of many colors of intaglio ink and the capabilities of the intaglio presses make it possible to achieve a different predominant color for each denomination with little increase over current production costs.

An alternative use of color to distinguish among denominations would be to apply color in a smaller area in a distinctive shape or coarse pattern (patterns are discussed in the following section). A small, distinctively placed patch of color would serve as an aid to orientation. The concept of distinctive denomination colors could possibly be combined with the large numeral by using the letter press to apply a single large numeral in color. The intaglio design would have to contain one large, clean area for application of any patch of color.

The letterpress, which applies the Treasury seal and the banknote serial number (in green) and the Federal Reserve Bank seal (in black), is used only on the front side of the banknote; it would be a major change to require two-side letterpress printing. In the current U.S. banknote design, the front side of the note is crowded, with the numerals and two seals occupying the majority of the space. There is little space for an additional colored mark anywhere on the banknote front. The Treasury and Federal Reserve Bank seals represent possible areas to color distinctively by denomination. Traditionally these seals are green and black, respectively. There may be restrictions on the colors that can be used for either of the seals.

The use of a predominant color for each denomination is useful to a large segment of the visually disabled population, including those whose visual acuity is below that required to read the denominational numerals, and there appear to be no technological impediments to implementation. The committee believes that this feature should be included in future banknotes.

Shapes and Coarse Patterns

Two additional visual features that have promise are the use of geometric shapes or coarse patterns to denote denomination. Geometric shapes (circles, squares, triangles, etc.) would preferably be large and printed on a clear or uncluttered background, just as the numerals would be (see Figure 4-2e). These sorts of shapes are currently in use on British currency (Jarvis, 1994). It would be necessary for users to learn the relationship between shape and note value. Since there is no logical connection between geometric shape and current note values, there would be some learning time necessary.

Coarse patterns are a variation of the above feature, except in this case, the position of this character (or characters) rather than the shape of the character determines note value. There may be a better intuitive connection here between the pattern of the characters and note value, and again, it would be very important to have large, high-contrast characters on an uncluttered background. Figure 4-2f depicts one example of the use of coarse patterns to aid in note denomination.

One subtlety to the coarse-pattern idea is that the printed pattern itself may be detailed (e.g., the portrait on the bill or a large unprinted watermark area) but may appear "coarse" to the person with low vision. The areas could be located at different, distinctive positions for the six denominations. Although people with low vision may not be able to identify the faces in portraits (or even see that they are faces), they may be able to use the locations of the patterns on the banknotes to gain information.

Any coarse features implemented must be large enough to be recognizable from a reasonable distance. While recognition of a large shape should not require as large a symbol as numeral recognition (discussed in Chapter 2), it is still reasonable to assume that patches the size of the Treasury and Federal Reserve Bank seals (with diameters approximately the same as the height of the current denomination numerals) would be difficult to identify for visually disabled people when viewed at a distance usual for cash transactions. As the committee recommends that numeral size should be larger than one-half the current banknote height to be legible for people with visual disabilities, it also recommends that any denominational shapes or coarse patterns used should be about the same size as the large numerals. The addition of color to these shapes or coarse patterns may improve their visibility and allow for smaller symbols to be used, since color recognition is generally easier than numeral or shape recognition.

The committee considers the shape feature to be secondary to large, high-contrast numerals with a uniform background or to denomination by color and believes that at best it would be a redundant clue for denomination. The coarse-pattern feature would be useful if the portraits or similar large, shaped patterns were distinctively located on the banknote.

TACTILE-ONLY FEATURES

Tactile features are those which rely on the sense of touch to provide information as to note denomination. At present the optimum height above the background and areal size of tactile features to give the best "readability" are not known. Braille dots are approximately 400 μm high; intaglio print can give a relief of 60–70 μm. Although research has been carried out on spacing of dots, limited results are available for actual relief perception and for the effect on perception of the interactions of feature area, shape height, etc. The French Post Office produced a stamp with embossed braille symbols 72 μm high. This was not easily readable by a committee member who is proficient in reading braille. It should be noted, however, that the task of identifying six denominations with a tactile mark is much less complex than the full character recognition required for braille markings. The difficulty in reading the stamp markings does not preclude the usefulness of tactile markings of this height for denominating banknotes. It does indicate that the tactile markings should be kept as simple as possible, with differentiation not depending on subtle differences between denomination symbols.

Several foreign countries have used different types of printed or embossed tactile marks on their banknotes with limited success (Koeze, 1990; Cruz V., 1994; Péterfi, 1994; Soekarna, 1994; Sirkis, 1994; Benali and Iraqi, 1994; Gaiteiro, 1994; Santipong, 1994; Johansen and Bjørgo, 1994; Trachsel and Meroni, 1994; Blomberg, 1994). Several of these sources mentioned that on crisp, new notes the printed tactile marks are quite readable, but marks quickly lose their distinctness with banknote wear, a fact that was confirmed by Koeze (1990). Nevertheless, tactile features potentially offer a variety of ways to assist visually disabled people in denominating banknotes if the durability problem is overcome.

Unlike the tactile features discussed above, there are other tactile features that involve the addition of information during paper manufacture or, alternatively, later in a printing or embossing operation. Features that could be incorporated during sheet manufacture include a tactile watermark and tactile threads or planchettes that would change the local thickness and thus could be detected by touch. The first feature is used in Japanese currency (Minoshima, 1994). A cross-section and a three-dimensional measurement of the watermark from a Japanese banknote are shown in Figure 4-3, indicating a depth of approximately 50 μm for the "doughnut-shaped" watermark (BEP, 1983). In any of the tactile marking cases, the number, frequency, or distribution of the perturbations could denote denomination.

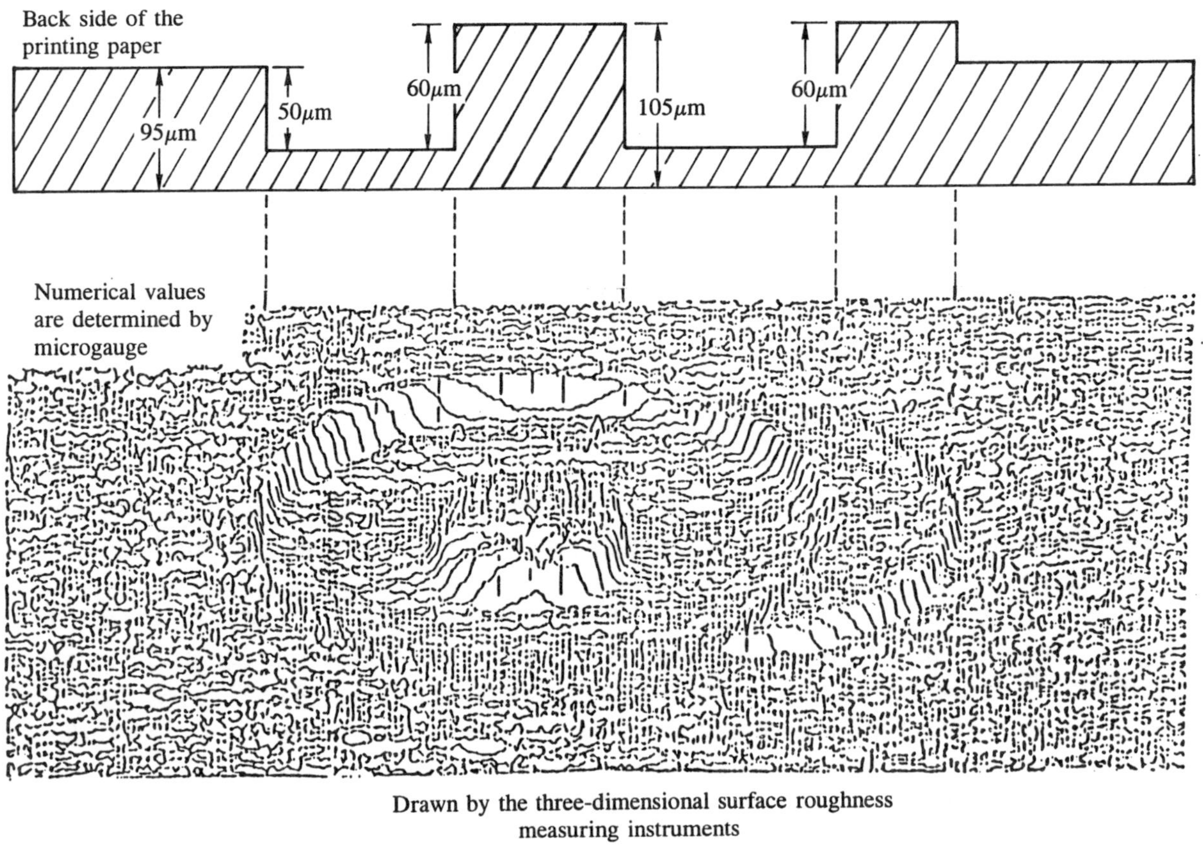

Figure 4-3 Illustration of variation in substrate thickness achieved by watermark in Japanese currency (BEP, 1983).

One major problem with most of these approaches is that stack height of the notes will be altered. This will always be the case with the addition of a local disturbance that increases sheet thickness. If such features always appear at the same location on the note, the bills may not stack evenly, causing a variety of problems for the BEP during manufacture and for the BEP, Federal Reserve banks, and other banks during subsequent handling. Many of the other countries using these types of features do not have the automated handling and stacking equipment used by the BEP and the Federal Reserve banks in the United States and so may not experience problems due to such markings.

One solution to the stacking problem is to not fix this feature to the same location on each note. However, this is generally an undesirable approach, since it adds complexity as the user does not know exactly where to look for the denomination clue. Another approach is to make the tactile information a negative displacement relative to the average thickness of the sheet. The tactile watermark uses this approach. Unfortunately, negative-displacement tactile information (holes or depressions) is much harder to "read" than positive displacement (bumps or points).

To avoid the above problems, the banknotes could include a texture that encompasses the entire surface area of a note. This "sandpaper" approach could be developed during the papermaking process or by embossing the paper after printing. An embossed surface that offered different patterns for different denominations could preserve stack "squareness," although stack height might differ from current height. However, if embossed patterns that would nest could be found, it might be possible to create stack heights that match the current ones. This possibility would make embossing an attractive option.

Changing sheet roughness during manufacture can be done, but there may not be enough of a range of tactile sensations to allow denomination of bills. Furthermore, the intaglio printing process would tend to flatten or smooth out the irregularities, as was found during the development of the Japanese watermark (Minoshima, 1994). A related approach would be to make the current substrate much smoother. This could accentuate the intaglio printing, making its tactile sensation more obvious or noticeable.

All of the tactile-only features discussed above will degrade with wear. Raised features, whether obtained by addition of specific materials or by embossing, will wear away, making the feature less useful. The tactile watermark is less prone to this type of degradation than printed or embossed features.

If the banknote base paper were a laminated structure, as is now the case for some security papers, it would be possible to punch holes in one of the outside lamination layers (illustrated in Figure 4-4). This could provide a negative tactile feature on one side while not compromising sheet strength or affecting stack height. Unfortunately, as noted in the discussion regarding holes, it is more difficult to "read" depressions (as compared with bumps). This means the depression caused by the hole in one ply of the laminated sheet, just like the tactile watermark, would probably not be a very effective aid for blind people.

The committee concludes here is that today there is no sure method to provide reliable tactile information on banknotes. The nature of research needed in this area is discussed in Chapter 5.

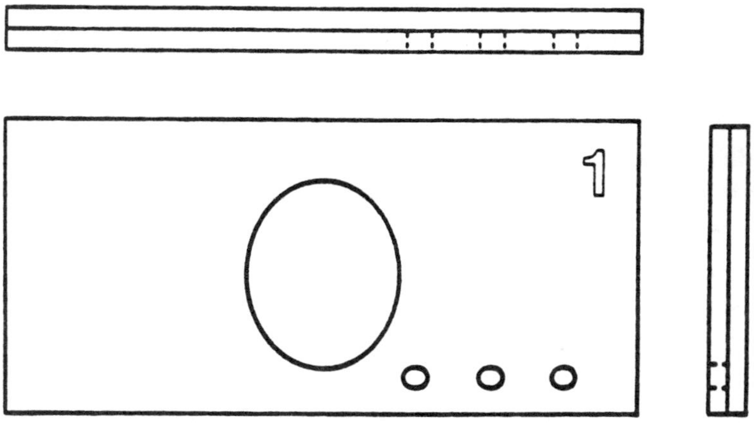

Figure 4-4 Holes in one thickness of a laminated structure.

MACHINE-READABLE FEATURES

This category includes features that can be used with devices that determine the denomination of a banknote. For a person who cannot benefit from visual security features, this is the only category of features that has the potential to authenticate the note, in addition to determining the denomination. Some of the features that would enhance the use of devices for denomination would be included in other categories, as they also give visual or tactile clues that can be read by an individual. Other features in this category are only useful with the aid of a device.

The previous sections have addressed the potential ways that visually disabled people could discriminate between different denominations without using devices. The committee strongly believes that these routes should be pursued as primary strategies, since the features suggested can be used without instrumental aids.

However, during the course of its discussions the committee concluded that the other three types of features (visual/tactile, visual-only, and tactile-only) did not provide a solution to the problem of banknote authentication. The committee felt that a device would provide the visually disabled community with a method of authentication. However, the committee also recognized that the principal device approach for blind people should be rapid denomination sorting, with the possibility of authentication where possible.

Potential devices form one area for future research; some concepts are discussed in Chapter 5. The current section addresses devices and features that would enhance device usability and that the committee felt were currently achievable and could therefore be addressed in the short term. The devices can be broken down into two categories: passive devices and active devices.

Passive Devices

In the section on visual/tactile features, the committee indicated that size differentiation among denominations could be a useful method of discrimination. This method could be made more reliable through the use of a simple size-guide template. Such a device is made with a fixed alignment corner and varying lengths and heights of notes given by a stepped opposite edge. The device can be made in many materials and be cheap enough to issue free through various agencies. This type of device may act as an educational aid to blind people in the early stages of implementation to give them confidence in their judgment on size-based discrimination. When a person becomes familiar with the new currency, the device may no longer be necessary.

Another feature discussed earlier in the report was holes. Various combinations and locations of holes could be used as a method of providing denomination discrimination. Again, a simple template would be useful. The template could contain notches that relate to the hole positioning and note values. Such a device was demonstrated to the committee (Oschwald and Hendricks, 1994).

Other examples of passive devices would be magnifying glasses, flashlights, etc., which would not be limited in usefulness to currency denomination.

Active Devices

In this category, the committee considered detection systems that require some basis of powered electronic analysis. Several banknote features that would enhance the use of these devices were considered.

Several of the features recommended in a previous National Research Council report (NRC, 1993) to discourage counterfeiting would enhance the ability of devices to denominate banknotes. Specifically, security threads with either width or location indicating denomination were recommended for incorporation in the near term and would allow device designers to design their equipment based on a known code. For intermediate- and long-term implementation, the optically active coated fibers and particles, as well as metallic or specular woven thread features, might be useful to designers of banknote denomination devices.

In addition to the features recommended in the previous report (NRC, 1993), the committee felt that a magnetic thread that contained a coding unique to each denomination could be inserted in the paper. This type of technology is known and has been incorporated in banknotes elsewhere, for example, in England and Italy.

A possibility exists to incorporate planchettes or fibers that contain machine-identifiable characteristics as opposed to the current red and blue fibers. By incorporating these planchettes or fibers in different volume distributions or banded locations, it should be possible to derive a code relating to the denomination. The principle of detection could be magnetic or radar/microwave. It is known that machine-identifiable fibers can be placed in banknote papers.

Since the use of uniform product code (UPC) or other coding is prevalent throughout the world, the committee considered the placement of an appropriate optical pattern code on the dollar bills. These codes would be specific to the denomination but not to the individual banknote. Many devices exist to read such codes, and they could form the basis for production of a small hand-held unit for blind people. The initial goal would be denomination sorting, as the committee recognizes that the code could be easily reproduced in a counterfeit manner. However, linkage with some other feature in the note could provide the basis for authentication. Dutch notes have this type of feature.

A feature that appears the same on both ends of the banknote would facilitate the design of devices that can denominate independent of note orientation. Examples of symmetrical features are ordinary barcodes that can be scanned in either direction, or a feature, such as a magnetic strip, that was located along the banknote length on the central axis.

The committee found that a number of countries throughout the world use fluorescent, magnetic, or infrared reactive inks. These inks could be incorporated in a simple bar code arrangement to allow for basic machine interrogation. These types of codes are used on Scottish banknotes and Eastern Caribbean Central Bank currency. Magnetic bar coding is used on the newer series of U.S. dollar bills and could be used as the basis for device design.

In the report based on the study conducted in 1983 by the BEP for U.S. Representative Edward Roybal, the BEP recommended continued development of electronic devices for denominating banknotes as the most effective way at that time to address the needs of the low vision and blind communities (BEP, 1983).

The committee was aware that Canada is currently promoting the use of a device to assist blind people in recognizing different denominations. It is estimated that there are almost 8,000 blind Canadians who cannot benefit from the large numerals and colors on the Canadian banknotes (Bank of Canada, 1994). Canadian currency designs contain colored patches approximately 4.75 mm square that indicate denomination by location and are interpreted by a device to provide denomination information. Since 1990, the Bank of Canada has supplied 4,600 readers (devices) free-of-charge to users through the Canadian National Institute for the Blind. There is a continued demand of about 50–60 readers per month. The readers are manufactured by Brytech Corporation and cost the Bank of Canada approximately $300 (Canadian) each. In a limited poll of users in 1991, the Bank of Canada determined that the majority of users are elderly and that they typically use the readers a few times a week at home, as opposed to carrying the readers with them as they work or shop. The Bank of Canada intends to conduct a more inclusive survey on the uses and usefulness of their readers and will work to improve the devices to make smaller or faster readers.

The committee feels that continued development of smaller and faster denomination devices will address the needs of people who are multiply handicapped or cannot otherwise use features available to denominate U.S. banknotes. Devices add a possibility of authentication for blind people, who cannot use the visual counterfeit-deterrent features. A way to help reduce the cost of designing and producing a denomination device is for the BEP to include one or more overt features in the new design that could be read by a device and interpreted for the user.

FEATURE COMBINATIONS

Combinations of features are likely to improve the ease with which banknotes can be denominated, as discussed in Chapter 2, and may also provide additional assistance in authentication (NRC, 1993). In addition, some combinations of features could improve the ability to distinguish front from back and to orient the face properly. Among the numerous possibilities might be dimensional changes combined with color, holes, or another tactile feature that would provide information regarding front-to-back and face orientation. Large numerals could be combined with color. Those combinations that also permit authentication and permit the inclusion of anticounterfeiting features should be favored.

Of the 171 banknote types described in the table in Appendix D, less than 40 percent are denominated using a single cue on each denomination; 28 use color only, and 31 use size only. Over 100 of the issuing authorities use both size and color on all denominations in the series, with some adding a tactile mark, large numerals, or both to increase the number of denominational cues available to visually disabled people. Four of these issuing authorities provide banknotes with color and a tactile symbol, so that there are two denominational cues.

The European Blind Union recommends that there be at least two different ways of discriminating among banknotes using two different senses (EBU, 1994). It is difficult to quantify the improvement in denomination ease with additional features, but complementary features add to the difficulty of simulation and might improve banknote security (NRC, 1993).

CONCLUSIONS AND RECOMMENDATIONS

From the long list of features that would assist in the denomination and authentication of banknotes, some were determined to be applicable immediately, some were dropped, and some would require investigation to determine if they are appropriate or if further research will make them applicable for currency use. Experience with some of the features is already available in other countries (Appendix D).

Visual/Tactile Features

The committee recommends the variation of length, height, or both dimensions as a key to denomination to address the needs of the broadest population. A secondary cue might provide orientation information. Aside from the use of devices, this feature is the only one that the committee recommends that addresses the needs of blind people.

The concept of holes for banknote denomination is attractive, but it is likely further from implementation than size variation. Although it would not be difficult to manufacture banknotes with holes in them, there are a number of issues regarding durability, public acceptance, etc., that require more work before this feature can be recommended for implementation.

Visual-Only Features

The committee recommends the use of large, high-contrast numerals on a simple, uniform background in the next redesign of U.S. banknotes. Incorporation of this feature would address the needs of a large fraction of the population for quick, easy identification of a banknote's denomination. The committee also recommends the use of different predominant colors for the six denominations printed. This feature addresses a large population as well and could be realized with little increase in unit costs. A third possibility, the use of geometric shapes and coarse patterns, is seen by the committee as a redundant, additional visual clue that might benefit the sighted but is not considered to be essential if the numerals are large enough and have sufficient background contrast.

Tactile-Only Features

The committee was unable to identify any tactile-only feature that can be recommended without further research.

Machine-Readable Features

The committee recommends the inclusion of overt features in the new currency design that would encourage the development of devices. Of the features considered, machine-detectable fibers, UPC coding, or simple geometric shapes in standard ink that could be read optically are readily available today. These same shapes in fluorescent, magnetic, or infrared inks might offer the possibility of lower-cost or smaller devices. The committee recommends that the Treasury Department and the Federal Reserve Bank work with the device developers to determine where the most improvements can be made.

Feature Combinations

As discussed in the Weber criteria section of Chapter 2, there are indications that combinations of features will be superior to any one by itself. These combinations tend to improve accuracy and to broaden the application range. Multiple features also may improve the ability to orient or authenticate a banknote.

REFERENCES

Abbott, G. 1994. Presentation to the Committee on Currency Features Usable by the Visually Impaired. March 1994.

Arditi, A. 1994. Presentation to the Committee on Currency Features Usable by the Visually Impaired. March 30, 1994.

Bank of Canada. 1994. Personal communication from Ms. M. Lefebvre-Manthorp of the Bank of Canada. July 8, 1994.

Benali, A., and M. Iraqi. 1994. Personal communication to the Committee on Currency Features Usable by the Visually Impaired. May 1994.

Bennett, D.G.M. 1994. Personal communication to the Committee on Currency Features Usable by the Visually Impaired. May 1994.

Blomberg, T. 1994. Personal communication to the Committee on Currency Features Usable by the Visually Impaired. May 1994.

Brabyn, J. A. 1994. Personal communication to the Committee on Currency Features Usable by the Visually Impaired. August 16, 1994.

BEP (Bureau of Engraving and Printing). 1983. A Study of Mechanisms for the Denomination of U.S. Currency by the Blind or Visually Impaired. Bureau of Engraving and Printing report to Congressman Edward R. Roybal, Chairman of the Select Committee on Aging, U.S. House of Representatives.

Church, S. 1994. Personal communication to the Committee on Currency Features Usable by the Visually Impaired. March 1994.

Cruz V., R. 1994. Personal communication to the Committee on Currency Features Usable by the Visually Impaired. June 1994.

Durlach N., L. Delhorne, A. Wong, W. Ko, W. Rabinowitz, and J. Hollerback. 1989. Manual discrimination and identification of length by the finger-span method. Perception and Psychophysics 46:29–38.

EBU (European Blind Union). 1994. A Report of the European Blind Union Expert Working Group on Currency: Recommendations for the Design of the ECU. Paris, France: EBU.

Farber, W. 1994. Personal communication to the Committee on Currency Features Usable by the Visually Impaired. May 1994.

Gaiteiro, J. 1994. Personal communication to the Committee on Currency Features Usable by the Visually Impaired. May 1994.

Hill, B.J. 1994. Presentation to the Committee on Currency Features Usable by the Visually Impaired. March 1994.

Jarvis, A. 1994. Personal communication to the Committee on Currency Features Usable by the Visually Impaired. May 1994.

Johansen, J. E., and J. Bjørgo. Personal communication to the Committee on Currency Features Usable by the Visually Impaired. May 1994.

King, S. 1994. Personal communication to the Committee on Currency Features Usable by the Visually Impaired. May 1994.

Koeze, P. 1990. A Large-Scale Experiment on the Effectiveness of the Marks for the Blind on Netherlands Banknotes. Presented at the European Banknote Printers' Conference, Rome.

Legge, G.E. 1994. Personal communication to the Committee on Currency Features Usable by the Visually Impaired. August 16, 1994.

Miller, O. 1994. Presentation to the Committee on Currency Features Usable by the Visually Impaired. March 1994.

Minoshima, Y. 1994. Personal communication to the Committee on Currency Features Usable by the Visually Impaired. May 1994.

National Research Council Committee on Vision. 1980. Recommended standard procedures for the clinical measurement and specification of visual acuity. Advances in Ophthalmology 41:103–148.

NRC (National Research Council). 1993. Counterfeit Deterrent Features for the Next-Generation Currency Design. National Materials Advisory Board, NRC. Washington, D.C.: National Academy Press.

Oschwald, J. and C. Hendricks. 1994. Presentation to the Committee on Currency Features Usable by the Visually Impaired. March 30, 1994.

Péterfi, S. 1994. Personal communication to the Committee on Currency Features Usable by the Visually Impaired. May 1994.

Santipong, C. 1994. Personal communication to the Committee on Currency Features Usable by the Visually Impaired. May 1994.

Sirkis, S. 1994. Personal communication to the Committee on Currency Features Usable by the Visually Impaired. May 1994.

Soekarna, E. 1994. Personal communication to the Committee on Currency Features Usable by the Visually Impaired. June 1994.

Trachsel, P., and M. Meroni. 1994. Personal communication to the Committee on Currency Features Usable by the Visually Impaired. May 1994.

Wallach, B. 1994. Presentation to the Committee on Currency Features Usable by the Visually Impaired. March 1994.

5

RESEARCH AND DEVELOPMENT NEEDS AND FUTURE DIRECTIONS

Considerable research work is underway on topics such as causes, degrees, and types of visual impairment; responses to tactile and visual stimuli; and devices to assist visually disabled people. These research and development programs have contributed significantly to an understanding of the needs of visually disabled people for participating fully in fundamental activities of life. Many of these research programs have resulted in approaches for meeting those needs. Although some of the understanding revealed by this work is applicable to the design of banknotes for visually disabled people, little of the technical work has specifically addressed the issue of banknote design and implementation. Essentially no research specifically addresses features that will make it possible for all visually disabled individuals to denominate U.S. banknotes independently and confidentially.

The research required covers three areas. The first is psychophysical, directed toward determination of the significant dimensions and gradation of steps that will permit reliable human discrimination of the features. The second level of research is practical materials science, which is directed toward the materials and processes that will yield durable, wear-resistant, survivable, and environmentally acceptable materials for printing features on, or for adding relief to, banknotes. The final area of research is applied science and engineering, which should have the intent of devising methods for economically and reliably imprinting the required features at a scale commensurate with the production of durable banknote features.

Two types of needs and directions require technical work. In the short term, there are features that are not technically difficult to incorporate, but optimization of these features is needed. The nature of the near-term studies will tend to be empirical and psychophysical. In the intermediate term, research is required to identify the thresholds and optimum application of low-relief features for tactile sensing. The research and development needs and directions for features that might be incorporated in the long term will be considerably more fundamental and require identification of appropriate physical characteristics of new features. The long-term research will, in many cases, be dependent on the potential applicability of developments in electronics, photonics, materials, and nanotechnology.

EMPIRICAL/PSYCHOPHYSICAL TECHNICAL NEEDS

As indicated in Chapter 4, the candidate features fall into a few categories. The technical information needed for features in each category is specified without detailed descriptions of research procedures. An organization undertaking to make the recommended measurements should be familiar with problems associated with visual impairment and proficient in performing the suggested determinations.

Visual/Tactile Features

Variable Dimensions

Most countries denominate banknotes by size along with other indicators. The size differences are generally in both length and width. The committee recommends thorough psychophysical studies to optimize the combination of length and height to permit reliable absolute judgment by banknote size. If a change in dimensions were to be made in U.S. banknotes, such knowledge would be helpful. Research in this area should be carried out with the goal of determining the optimum strategy for implementing the size variations recommended in Chapter 4.

In some instances, templates are supplied to ensure that blind people will be able to denominate banknotes in accordance with size differences. In countries where templates have been supplied, it has been observed that after a short time, people who are blind learn to recognize denominations utilizing their sense of touch and no longer use the templates. On the other hand, if templates were built into wallets or other types of billfolds, it is probable that they would be used much more extensively. Such an arrangement would be of great help to those whose sense of touch has been impaired later in life, such as individuals with advanced cases of diabetes.

Holes

A practical concern is the effect of hole shape, size, number, and spacing on durability and wear. Empirical tests that address such questions are very much in order. It is important to determine the optimum hole size for easy identification and for rigidity with wear. Given an optimum hole size, the number and locations that are required to ensure accurate denomination and orientation would need to be determined. The effectiveness of the combination of a single hole for orientation or denomination with banknote dimensional changes for denomination should be assessed in terms of durability, wear, reliability, and aesthetics.

The wear characteristics of suitable holes would need to be determined. Materials and processes appropriate for edging and forming such holes need to be identified. The treatment of the edges of such holes to promote long-term durability is an area that requires more research.

Some research is also needed into the willingness of the public to accept banknotes that contains marks generally interpreted as invalidating.

Visual-Only

There is substantial literature on visual processes and perception under a range of conditions. The committee found that most of the data are not directly relevant to the specific case of banknote applications. Identification of the smallest useful set of features should be made, and optimum use of these features identified. One or more colors could easily be combined with a visual/tactile feature or with a feature that is tactile only. Early research into these features should establish a basis for contrast, size of features, and selection of appropriate colors that can be used to enhance discrimination by visually disabled persons. The existence of an extensive visual science literature indicates that identification of requisite characteristics of these features would require development, not research.

Numerals

Though there is a substantial body of research on size (width and height) of characters; optimum optical contrast as a function of illumination, intensity, and wavelength; whether the characters should be black on white or the converse; optimum location; and whether characters should be in more than one location, there has been little research directed toward banknote denomination and recognition. Application of the existing body of research to the optimum type of numerals and ratio of numeral-to-background areas for banknote denomination requires some development, and continued research into more long-term ideas, such as the effectiveness of fluorescence or scintillation in the areas occupied by the numerals, is recommended.

Color

The selection of effective colors for banknote denomination, as well as the degree of saturation required to ensure easy and accurate recognition by visually disabled individuals, is an area about which much is still unknown. To maximize color discrimination over as wide a range of lighting conditions as possible, development is needed on the application of color theory to the selection of hues for banknote denomination.

Included in this effort should be optimum colored area, size, location, number, shape, and color combinations. It is also possible to incorporate phosphorescent or fluorescent material that would glow if illuminated by ultraviolet light or in some cases by ordinary white light. Such an attribute may be extremely useful under poor illumination conditions for normally sighted individuals as well. One or more counterfeit deterrents could also be incorporated in colored areas.

Optically variable inks are being considered in the new banknote design. Research is needed to determine if this feature would be applicable to denomination coding of banknotes or if it is too subtle for people with low vision.

Tactile-Only

If tactile-only features were to be incorporated into banknotes, certain information about the nature of such features is essential in order to maximize the probability that they will be useful over the life of the banknote. There is some question about whether the raised areas should be bumps; characters; lines; or some other shape, such as a doughnut. Information on minimum height to ensure accurate, reliable recognition is essential, as is the effect of age and wear as a function of height. The optimum presentation of a tactile mark needs to be approached in terms of banknote manufacturing, as well as the psychophysical or human factors area.

Most research in tactile character reading has concentrated on braille, where the symbols are approximately 400 μm higher than the background surface. In contrast, intaglio printing can produce features approximately 60–70 μm high. Short-term investigations into ability to read such low-relief features should establish minimum detectable feature heights and dimensions. The nature of the tactile feature, that is, its shape; the number of individual elements (such as dots or lines); and the spacing of any individual elements will have an effect on the minimum detectable height and need to be considered in concert with the height criteria. Knowing minimum detectable feature heights and dimensions would allow researchers to determine the acceptable amount of wear that a tactile feature can experience before the feature is no longer useful.

To ensure that these tactile marks remain recognizable over the lifetime of the banknote, more-durable marks than are currently available will be required. More investigation into methods of making the tactile marks durable is necessary before implementation can be recommended.

Another problem that would require research is the effect of raised or tactile features on the ability to manufacture, stack, and sort banknotes at high speed and to determine what sorts of tactile features would minimize these problems.

There has been extensive research into the most effective way to present tactile denominators, especially in the Netherlands. The committee recommends that the Treasury Department and the Federal Reserve stay apprised of the work going on overseas and of experiences with circulation of banknotes with various types of tactile marks.

As a result of the technical work discussed, raised-relief features could be developed and tested against sound technical guidelines.

Feature Combinations

Research is recommended to study various combinations of features to determine an optimum set to improve ease of denomination or to add authentication or orientation information. The extent of success of visually disabled individuals in using these combinations should be quantified, and the research carried out in this area should be directed toward the identification of a figure of merit for combinations of features.

Substrate Materials

For several of the features discussed to be more effective and more durable, research is needed on the currency base paper. The fibrous composition and sizing of this substrate is specified by the government and has changed little through the years. Research that could lead to greater durability and thus longer life even in current banknotes would be beneficial. It would be appropriate to consider other, new fiber furnishes (containing some portion of synthetic fibers, for example) or layered composite structures. Some synthetic (plastic) papers may also be suitable as currency base paper.

A composite substrate that could resist abrasion would be ideal for tactile features to aid visually disabled as well as normally sighted people. Tactile features might also be more effective with the use of a smoother substrate, from which they would stand out more easily.

Current paper-making practices result in papers that delaminate easily, usually because the hydrodynamic forces during paper making cause the fibers to be arranged in the plane of the sheet with very little out-of-plane orientation. A substrate that would resist delamination, perhaps a composite in which the fibers had some out-of-plane orientation or contained tough synthetic fibers, would be ideal for banknote features involving holes, clipped corners, or modified edges. Research directed to improve current U.S. banknote base paper could have significant impact on note durability and on the ability to incorporate certain counterfeiting deterrents, as well as robust aids to help visually disabled people.

Devices

The committee agrees that a desirable approach would be to permit virtually all visually disabled individuals, together with normally sighted persons, to denominate banknotes without the aid of devices. It is conceivable, however, that under certain circumstances very simple, inexpensive, unobtrusive, and accurate devices could be of assistance under dim lighting conditions—not only to visually disabled people but also to normally sighted individuals.

Since a device is the only method of authentication of banknotes by a blind individual, it is appropriate for short-term technical work to be undertaken that concerns itself with the potential advantages and utility of very simple devices that could be available immediately. Together with this should be a longer-term, highly focused research and development program designed to derive much more sophisticated devices.

Adaptation of Current Devices

Fixed-placement devices are currently in use in vending machines, ATMs, and retail establishments (e.g., ultraviolet lamps to detect the presence of optical brighteners). Information should be provided on overt features to enable device designers to make devices more portable, smaller, faster, and more reliable, both for use by visually disabled individuals and for those who currently use fixed-placement devices.

Some types of very simple, inexpensive, devices that are currently available and that could prove useful for banknote denomination in various settings are a small flashlight on a key chain, which could be made wavelength-selective utilizing filters; a small magnifying glass, perhaps equipped with a light source; plastic templates that could be used to denominate different-sized banknotes (were there a hole in the currency, this template could also be used for front-to-back differentiation and rotational orientation); a light source such as either light-emitting diodes (LEDs) or lasers to emit a single wavelength or a broad spectrum of light; and finally, a very simple magnetometer that senses a predetermined magnetic pattern in the banknote and converts the information to aural, visual, or tactile information. In all cases, the physical processes are well known, but research and development into miniaturization and reliability is required. It is likely that such development will be market driven.

Technologically Advanced Devices

Very advanced devices could not only recognize and denominate but also authenticate banknotes. They must be inexpensive, reliable, easy to use, inconspicuous, and quick, and they must give acceptable rates of false positive and false negative readings. Ideally, such a device would be built into a wallet or other equally ordinary item and provide a visual, aural, or tactile response. Devices of this kind would probably require incorporation of active or passive material into bank notes. The possibilities are myriad. However, the performance and cost requirements are extraordinarily stringent.

It is highly probable that the basic technology on which such devices will be predicated will come from significant advances in areas like photonics, molecular electronics, microwave and radar emission and sensing, microelectronics, nanotechnology, and materials. Research in these areas is increasingly underway in university, government, and industrial research and development laboratories. For example, low-cost radar technology developed at the Lawrence Livermore National Laboratories has been adapted for use in inexpensive tools that permit location of wires, pipes, and studs in walls and underground (FLC, 1994). Another possibility could be based on an LED array and a photosensor. Such a device could be very small and, with continued materials and manufacturing advances, quite inexpensive. In addition to staying abreast of the research and development discussed, it is also imperative for currency designers and manufacturers to maintain contact with the research and development centers concerned with aiding visually disabled people.

It is important that advances in the various potentially relevant sciences and engineering disciplines be monitored and their relevance to potential Treasury Department or BEP interests or needs recognized. The committee supports the approach suggested in the National Research Council report on anticounterfeiting measures that the BEP or other appropriate body sponsor annual or semi-annual technical workshops (NRC, 1993), in this case to encourage development of the field of features usable by visually disabled people.

Smart Money

The long-range possibility that features can be developed that will permit individuals with any degree of visual impairment to both denominate and authenticate banknotes cannot be ignored. Such currency might respond to touch and transmit to the individual aural, visual, or tactile information that would permit easy, rapid denomination and authentication. The principal barrier would probably not be technology but the development of durable materials and the cost of manufacturing. The components might be divided into two parts, with the very inexpensive portion incorporated in the note and the more expensive portion built into a very simple, easy-to-use aid such as a wallet or a card or glove. These types of designs may prove to be too expensive for inclusion in lower denominations but could be used effectively in larger denomination banknotes.

CONCLUSIONS AND RECOMMENDATIONS

Development of features building on the extensive literature on visual and tactile processes and perception is warranted for near-term banknote feature additions. Highly directed, psychophysical/empirical technical work should be undertaken as a high priority effort that addresses questions regarding optimum dimensions, optical contrast, location, colors, physical size, etc., for making recognition and denomination of U.S. banknotes easy, convenient, and inconspicuous for visually disabled individuals.

Similar to the work suggested for individual banknote features, technical work should also be performed to identify combinations of features that enhance denomination and orientation.

Near- or mid-term research is required to define the threshold and accuracy for reading the types of low-relief tactical features that are likely to be applicable to banknotes. Long-term research into advanced features, possibly leading to smart money, should be initiated as possible directions become evident from technology development.

Advances in microelectronics, nanotechnology, molecular electronics, materials, photonics, and magnetics should not only be followed but also encouraged by supporting technical work that is focused on deriving very sophisticated but inexpensive, reliable, accurate, inconspicuous devices to assist visually disabled people in recognizing, denominating, and perhaps authenticating U.S. banknotes.

Technical work underway by organizations and institutions concerned with the problems of people who are visually disabled and with solutions to those problems should also be followed. Very often, these organizations themselves maintain contact with the technological areas identified and are in a position to adapt them for their own purposes, that is, to ultimately benefit visually disabled individuals.

REFERENCES

FLC. 1994. FLC Newslink. June.

NRC (National Research Council). 1993. Counterfeit Deterrent Features for the Next-Generation Currency Design. National Materials Advisory Board, NRC. Washington, D.C.: National Academy Press.

6

IMPLEMENTATION STRATEGIES

If denomination features are to be incorporated into U.S. banknotes, the major objectives of the implementation strategy should be to ensure that:

- those features incorporated become available in a timely and cost-effective manner;
- the new banknotes can cocirculate with the old;
- counterfeit-deterrent features already present in the new banknotes or planned for the near future are not compromised by the additional features; and
- an adequate and extensive public education program is undertaken, so that all visually disabled individuals and the general public learn how to use these new features.

Introduction of the new design will begin with the issue of the new $100 bill by 1996, which will be followed by designs for the lower denominations at a rate of approximately one denomination design per year (Church, 1994). As stated by representatives of the Treasury Department and BEP when they introduced the new banknote design (see Appendix F), each denomination banknote in a sequence does not need to have all the same features, either for counterfeit deterrence or for denomination by visually disabled people. In this case, features that the committee recommends for intermediate-term implementation (three to five years) may be incorporated within the current redesign sequence. In addition to the current redesign effort, in the future banknote designs will be changed at more frequent intervals than they have been previously, mostly to deter counterfeiting resulting from rapidly improving technology. By the time of the next redesign of the $100 banknote, features that are recommended for long-term research may have matured to the point of implementation.

The BEP may choose to include features that are more expensive to implement only in the higher denomination banknotes, even though the technology is currently available. For example, the polyester security thread introduced in the 1990 series of banknotes is not expected to be incorporated into the $1 bill because of its cost. It would, however, be worthwhile to ensure the encorporation of some features in the more frequently used banknotes (the lower denominations).

FEATURE IMPLEMENTATION

This subsection has been divided into three parts. The first deals with features that can be implemented in a very short time because they require only psychophysical determinations and field testing. The second concerns those features that require some technological development that would be followed by psychophysical studies and field tests. The third treats features that cannot be implemented given the current state of worldwide technology. Advanced and fundamental research and development must be successfully completed before serious consideration of such a feature would be possible.

Near Term (1 to 3 Years)

Some features, such as dimensional changes, large numerals, and appropriate use of color, can be incorporated into the present currency redesign. Other features, such as denominational holes, can be added to near-term banknote changes in a orderly manner without unduly delaying currency redesign and issuance.

Dimensional Changes

The technology required to produce banknotes that are sized differently depending on denomination is very well known and widely used. By choosing the most frequently printed banknote, the $1 bill, to be the smallest, there will be savings in the cost of materials that may well offset the increase in cost of capital investment and additional operations required for producing a set of graded size currencies, as discussed in Chapter 4.

Implementation of this feature would require careful planning and a great deal of notification about upcoming changes for all who are involved in the design or manufacture of cash-handling machines. For example, the sorting machines at the Federal Reserve and commercial currency dispensing and reading machines will have to be altered. The widespread use of machines in Europe capable of handling a variety of national currencies indicates that this alteration would not be a technical problem and might be accomplished through the natural periodic replacement of currency machines. If two-dimensional size changes are not to be used, a possible implementation strategy might be to change only the length of the banknote with denomination. Since banknote height is more critical for machine handling than banknote length, this strategy should minimize the impact of a size change on the variety of cash-handling machines.

As always, there are other issues that need to be considered. U.S. banknotes have been the same size for at least 65 years, and there may, therefore, be a reluctance on the part of the population to change. On the other hand, U.S. coins are very easy to differentiate, because their size, feel, composition, edge treatment, and color are all different. Acceptance of this size differentiation in coins is complete by the American population and so, with sufficient preparation, might be acceptance of a change to size-denominated banknotes. Education of the public about the reasons for the size changes and the benefits of having size-denominated banknotes would help the population accept the inconveniences associated with this change.

With size-denominated banknotes there is the possibility of using a template or guide to learn the size/denomination code. In the early stages of distributing sized banknotes, these templates must be readily available, so a part of the implementation strategy for this feature should include the distribution of appropriate templates. The templates should be distributed free of charge, through the banks, as in England, or through other appropriate organizations, as in Canada. The potential for using such devices to advertise products or services should also be considered.

Holes

The technology for producing holes in paper is well known and often used outside the banknote production community. The capital equipment expenditure required, though not zero, is minimal. One of the significant potential advantages of holes is broad applicability, that is, across all visually disabled and normally sighted people. There are a number of psychological and traditional issues associated with putting holes into banknotes that were identified previously in this report. Education about the use and benefits of this feature would play a large part in its successful introduction.

Another major implementation issue with using holes to denominate, whether by number of holes, hole shape, or hole location, would be cocirculation of banknotes containing this feature and older banknotes without holes. The possibility of punching holes in an old series $1 bill to imitate a $20 banknote of the new series cannot be overlooked, and a strategy to prevent this type of "raising" must accompany the introduction of the feature. The banknotes with the new design must contain another, less-counterfeitable feature to enable people who are blind to distinguish between the older and the newer banknotes. This accompanying feature may only serve to distinguish the new design banknotes from the older ones and does not need to contain any denomination information. For example, a tactile mark may be found that maintains enough distinction over the life of a banknote to serve as a "go/no go" indicator; the presence of this tactile mark would indicate that the banknote is of the new design and that the hole-denomination cue is appropriate.

Large, High-Contrast Numerals

The technology for producing numerals that are large and have high contrast is known. It would be relatively inexpensive to incorporate large numerals into the banknote design, and there is little or no capital equipment expenditure required. The issues are those of design, as the large numerals must be of high contrast against an uncluttered background in order to be effective for the largest number of visually disabled people. Very little education for the public would be necessary for this feature.

The size and optical contrast of the numerals should be such that denomination is possible at a reasonable distance by people who are visually disabled so that their transactions are as effortless as those performed by normally sighted individuals. Large numerals with a highly contrasting background could be used to incorporate anticounterfeiting features, as long as the high contrast is maintained on a macroscopic scale. Such features should be incorporated into the overall banknote design in such a way as to minimize distraction from other security features in the banknote.

Color

As in the case of large numerals, the technology to implement this feature is well known; it can be inexpensive and easy to implement, and it does not require fundamental changes in the BEP's method of producing currency and capital equipment. The major technical decisions would be the selection of colors and the choice of appropriate inks. As with size-denominated banknotes, the most important implementation strategy should focus on public education.

Denomination Aids

Promotion of some of the types of devices mentioned in Chapter 5 (in the section on "Adaptation of Current Devices") by the issuing authorities should accompany the introduction of any visual-only features.

Intermediate Term (Three to Five Years)

Two types of features fit this category. One of them would be based on purely tactile features, and the other on devices that have some form of aural, visual, or tactile output.

Tactile-Only

As indicated in the previous chapters, a great deal appears to be unknown about the efficacy of tactile dots, lines, and entire characters in assisting visually disabled individuals to read the information. Assuming that the questions are resolved, implementation of these features will require the appropriate investment in equipment by the BEP. For either embossed or printed tactile features, as with holes, older banknotes without the feature could be modified to appear as if it were a newer banknote of higher denomination containing the feature. Again, implementation of these types of features would require that there be an independent method of distinguishing older-design banknotes from the newer-design ones.

Printed transparent-ink tactile marks could be added in areas not occupied with intaglio printing. The amount of design change necessary to get a fully effective feature will depend on the design chosen but need not be great. Because of the minimal impact on design, the timing of this feature's incorporation is potentially flexible. If this feature is deemed to be effective after investigation, invisible tactile marks could be added to banknotes as the technology becomes available without major alterations in the banknote design.

Devices

Means for reading magnetic, conductive, and optical patterns instrumentally are well established, as is the technology required to convert the resulting electronic signals to aural, visual, or tactile information recognizable by the user. Such a device could also authenticate banknotes if enough sophistication were built into it. It is highly probable that, as such devices are improved, among the first uses would be point-of-sale applications, especially for blind or visually disabled individuals employed in positions that require them to handle currency on a daily basis. It would be desirable for all devices to accept and denominate banknotes independent of banknote orientation.

Although the market for portable devices will ultimately be fairly large, it will probably not be considered a mass market for some time. The Treasury Department or BEP should consider working with device designers so that both the sensor technology and the banknote features are developed in parallel, enabling implementation of the full system with one design change.

Long Term (More Than Five Years)

It is virtually impossible to predict what technical advances in microelectronics, nanotechnology, materials and molecular electronics will make possible in the next few years, much less in more than five years. Therefore, staying abreast of advances in these areas and related ones and keeping in mind the related functions and characteristics that future banknote designs should satisfy appears to be the only feasible approach.

One possibility that the committee considered is a banknote that has the built-in capability to indicate denomination by itself, sometimes referred to as "smart money." Such indication could be aural, visual, or tactile and could respond to a direct user stimulus such as touch. Implementation is very long range and dependent on a myriad of technical advances.

FIELD TESTING

The results of the psychophysical technical work recommended in the previous chapter would indicate optimum characteristics of individual features and likely combinations. However, true effectiveness can only be determined by those who would ultimately use these features. The Treasury Department and Federal Reserve should involve appropriate user groups as early as possible to ensure selection of those features most likely to be used by, and useful to, the target population.

New currency design is generally carried out with a high level of confidentiality. This confidentiality can be maintained in appropriate field test design by separate testing of individual features. Even though broadly based field tests utilizing all classes of visually disabled individuals are not practical, some evaluations in "real life" situations prior to introduction of new currency features are mandatory. The many organizations that represent people who are blind and people with various types of visual impairment represent a resource for performing limited field tests on a confidential basis. The test conditions should be as close as possible to everyday uses of currency but can be targeted to the evaluation of a single feature rather than the entire banknote design. The field test should be broad enough in scope to show that the new feature permits rapid, relatively effortless, and confidential banknote denomination under not only optimal conditions but also across a wide range of everyday circumstances.

The nature of such tests and the means of handling the statistical data should be assigned to independent experts skilled in conducting such studies. The resulting data, combined with the results of the psychophysical investigations, can then be used to develop specifications for each feature that designers responsible for ultimately incorporating them will have to satisfy. The results of this type of testing could also be used to determine the extent and content of public education that will be needed for successful introduction of the tested feature. The analysis should include determining whether the banknote feature introduction will reduce the security of banknote use by visually disabled people. Any reduction in security, especially during the introductory phase of new banknotes, also needs to be addressed in the public education campaign.

CONCLUSIONS AND RECOMMENDATIONS

- Technologies are available now to include size denomination; large, high contrast numerals; and the use of color to denote denomination.
- Because of the current redesign schedule, it will be three to five years before the lower-denomination banknotes will be designed and produced. This schedule will make it possible to incorporate into those banknotes features that must still undergo some development and field testing (for example, durable tactile markings). Because banknote redesign can be anticipated on a more frequent cycle than in the past, the opportunity will return to redesign the higher denominations, in which features recommended for long-term research (e.g., "smart money") might be considered.
- Some features will not be cost-effective for inclusion in the design of lower-denomination banknotes, even though the technology to produce those banknotes is available today. However, features should be made available in the most frequently used banknotes (the lower denominations).
- For any of the features proposed, successful implementation would require a large public education program. The particulars of the program will depend on the features incorporated and can be determined from the results of field testing done prior to incorporation of the feature on a banknote.
- Cocirculation with older banknotes will be a problem for features that are basically a slight modification to the present design and can be easily simulated or added by a counterfeiter, such as punched holes. For these features, there must be another, less easily simulated feature implemented at the same time that will distinguish the new series banknotes from the older ones, although it might not necessarily carry denominational information itself.
- Tactile features printed with transparent ink can be implemented with minimal design changes and so offer some flexibility in timing the feature incorporation.
- It is highly likely that the types of auxiliary denomination devices suggested for the intermediate term (three- to five-year period) will be developed. However, there appears to be some question about whether the size and cost objectives for convenient denomination devices can be met in this short period of time. It is therefore likely that the first use and mass market

will be for point-of-sale applications. The income from this market may very well encourage manufacturers to undertake the research and development required to substantially reduce size and cost.

REFERENCES

Church, S. 1994. Personal communication from Sara Church, BEP, to the Committee on Currency Features Usable by the Visually Impaired.

7

RECOMMENDATIONS

Throughout the report, a number of recommendations are made.[1] Foremost are features for visually disabled people that the committee believes could be incorporated in the redesigned currency currently under development by the New Currency Design Task Force. Other recommendations include strategies for the field testing of features and implementation strategies for features incorporated in the new design to enhance the effectiveness of the features and to educate the public in their use. In the opinion of the committee, some of the features identified in this report as potentially useful for visually disabled people could be incorporated without significant further research.

Since advances in reproduction and imaging technologies will require more-frequent redesign of the currency to combat counterfeiting, the committee has identified areas where further research may broaden the range of features applicable to the denomination, identification, and authentication of currency and enhance the effectiveness of the features recommended.

RECOMMENDED FEATURES

- The committee recommends the use of size as a key to denomination, with or without the use of a size template (4).
- The committee suggests evaluation of current approaches to size-denominated currency in other countries and determination of the magnitude of size differences that would make the six denominations sufficiently distinguishable (4).
- The committee strongly recommends the use of large, high-contrast numerals on a uniform background (4).
- The committee recommends the use of different predominant colors for the six denominations printed (4).
- The committee considers coarse features to be secondary to the use of large, high-contrast numerals with a uniform background or color. These features would be useful if the portraits or other similar large, shaped patterns were distinctively located on the banknote (4).

[1] The number in parentheses at the end of each recommendation refers to the chapter in the body of the report where the recommendation is discussed.

- The committee recommends that some overt features be included in the new currency design to assist the developers of devices. Of the features considered, denominational UPC coding or simple geometric shapes included in the intaglio design in standard ink could be read optically and are readily available today (4).
- Specification of new or enhanced features should not be aimed at minimal levels of recognition performance (i.e., threshold levels) but should strive for sufficient differentiation to permit rapid, effortless performance. Differences between successive denominations should be several times larger than the difference threshold (2).

RESEARCH AND DEVELOPMENT OPPORTUNITIES

- Development of features building on the extensive literature on visual and tactile processes and perception is warranted for near-term currency feature additions. Highly directed, psychophysical/empirical technical work should be undertaken to address questions regarding optimum dimensions, optical contrast, location, colors, physical size, etc. (5).
- The committee recommends research to define the threshold and accuracy of reading of the types of low-relief tactile features that are likely to be applicable to currency. This information would be needed for assessment of tactile features should a technique be identified for production of appropriate durable tactile marks (5).
- The committee urges research on the development of durable tactile features printed with transparent ink, since they can be implemented with minimal design changes and so offer flexibility in timing the feature incorporation (6).
- The committee recommends that combinations of features that enhance denomination and orientation be identified (5).
- The committee recommends research on enhanced threads or planchettes that would improve the use of devices (4).
- The committee recommends that the Treasury Department, the Federal Reserve, and the BEP work with the device developers to determine where the most improvements can be made (4).
- The committee recommends that long-term research into advanced features, possibly leading to smart money, be initiated as possible directions become evident from technology development (5).
- The committee recommends that the incorporation of advances in microelectronics, nanotechnology, molecular electronics, materials, photonics, and magnetics in device development be encouraged by supporting technical work that is focused on deriving very sophisticated but inexpensive, reliable, accurate, and inconspicuous devices to assist visually disabled people in recognizing; denominating; and, perhaps, authenticating U.S. currency (5).
- Technical work underway by organizations and institutions concerned with the problems of people who are visually disabled and with solutions to those problems should be followed (5).

IMPLEMENTATION STRATEGIES

- In selecting features for implementation, the Treasury Department and the Federal Reserve should involve appropriate user groups as early as possible to ensure selection of those features most likely to be used by, and useful to, the target population (6).
- The field test should be broad enough in scope to show that the new feature permits rapid, relatively effortless, and confidential currency identification not only under optimal conditions but across a wide range of everyday circumstances (6).
- Data gathered from focus groups should be used to help guide the public education campaign that must be a part of the implementation of any new currency feature (6).
- Should graded sizes of currency be introduced, the introduction schedule would have to follow modifications of the BEP's production equipment and allow some period of time for the commercial currency-handling industry to prepare for the change (6).
- In the early stages of distributing sized currency, templates must be made readily available, so a part of the implementation strategy for this feature must include the distribution of appropriate templates. The templates should be distributed free of charge, using banks or appropriate organizations of and for visually disabled people (6).

APPENDIX A: EXECUTIVE SUMMARY IN LARGE PRINT

There are an estimated 3.7 million people in the United States who are visually disabled, that is, who have corrected visual acuity no better than 20/70[1] in the better eye or who have a maximum visual field of no more than 30 degrees (Genensky, 1994). About 200,000 of these people are blind (have no useful pattern vision), and 3.5 million have low vision. The leading causes of low vision are diseases that are common in old age: age-related maculopathy, cataract, glaucoma, diabetic retinopathy, and optic nerve atrophy. Almost 10 percent of the population 75 to 84 years of age experiences low vision, while 25 percent of the population 85 and older is deemed to have low vision. Yet, low vision is not confined to the old; an estimated 1 million persons below age 65 experience low vision, and 72 thousand under 65 are blind (Genensky, 1994). An additional 9 million Americans live with other, milder forms of visual impairment that interfere with daily living tasks, especially in adverse lighting conditions (Benson and Marano, 1994).

---

[1] There are a variety of ways to define levels of visual acuity. One common definition is to find the smallest letters a person can read at a standard distance (traditionally, 20 feet) and express the result as the ratio of this distance to the distance at which a "normal" observer can read the same letters. (In the case cited, the "normal" observer could read the specified letters at 70 feet, hence, acuity of 20/70.)

An important aspect of a person's full participation in today's society is being able to conveniently and confidentially exchange currency in everyday transactions, as when using public transportation or making purchases (EBU, 1994). U.S. citizens with low vision experience a uniquely difficult task in that U.S. banknotes are remarkably uniform in size, color, and general design. The banknotes provide no basis for denominating by blind persons. Visual identification of denomination by people with low vision is generally so challenging that many revert to techniques used by people who are blind.

Blind people must trust others to inform them about the denominations of bills received. In the absence of features that are usable by blind people in the present bills, different denominations, once identified by a trusted sighted person, are sorted and stored in different ways.

FEATURES IN USE WORLDWIDE

The committee has identified 171 issuing authorities in the world producing banknotes. Many have specifically addressed the problems of people with low vision by incorporating such features as variable size, variable color, and tactile markings. In some cases, a device is made available to blind people to aid in denominating banknotes. For example, England issues a size template, and Canada supplies its blind citizens with a portable banknote reader with audio output.

NEW BANKNOTE DESIGN

By 1996, the U.S. Treasury Department's Bureau of Engraving and Printing (BEP) expects to begin production of a new design for the $100 bill. In each succeeding year, working in descending order, a new design for a denomination will be introduced. By the year 2001, all six denominations currently in production ($100, $50, $20,

$10, $5, and $1) will have been redesigned. A major motivation for this redesign is the incorporation of new security features to combat the threat of counterfeiting posed by the rapid development in advanced copying and imaging systems that allow even the unskilled user to make faithful full-color reproductions of documents.

This redesign presents an opportunity to introduce features into the design that will make U.S. banknotes more readily usable by visually disabled people. The timetable of the redesign also presents the opportunity to incorporate features that may require some development work into the smaller denominations within the current redesign sequence. To this end, the Committee on Currency Features Usable by the Visually Impaired was charged to:

- assess features that could be used by people who are visually disabled to recognize, denominate, and authenticate banknotes;
- recommend features that could reasonably be incorporated into banknotes using available technology;
- suggest strategies that should be instituted to make the recommended features most effective; and
- identify research needs in particularly promising areas that could lead to attractive future approaches.

In the study, three aspects of currency transactions were defined: recognition (is this meant to be a banknote?), denomination (how much is it worth?), and authentication (is it a real banknote?). An additional consideration of importance, especially with regard to the use of machines accepting cash, was the usefulness of features indicating orientation of the banknote. The primary goal of the committee was to recommend features that will help visually disabled people denominate banknotes, since reliable denomination is essential to their maintaining independence. The committee also evaluated features that will help these individuals authenticate banknotes, a process for which the individuals have the same needs as the normally sighted public. Such features could be added in addition to those included for use in denomination. The committee did not consider the entire mix of the circulating medium in the U.S. but focused solely on solutions to problems dealing with banknotes.

FEATURE ASSESSMENT CONSIDERATIONS

Over the course of this study, the committee solicited presentations from experts in visual and tactile perception and from representatives of organizations of blind people and people with low vision. The committee also obtained considerable data on currency features usable by visually disabled people and incorporated in the currency of other countries.

The committee generated an extensive list of features representing a wide range of sensory phenomena and application technologies. In assessing and prioritizing these features, the committee used an approach similar to that taken for the evaluation of counterfeit-deterrent features for currency in a previous study (NRC, 1993). In this approach, the set of requirements for a feature was converted into indicators or criteria that were considered in terms of relative importance. The application of the feature to different target populations was considered. Features of use to the broadest range of people were ranked highest.

The criteria for banknote feature effectiveness were first divided into target and evaluation criteria. The target population categories were blind, low vision, normally sighted in adverse lighting, and normally sighted in normal lighting. While visually disabled people were the primary group to be considered in regard to the features, normally sighted people would also benefit from any features implemented. The target function categories were recognition, denomination, authentication, and orientation. Orientation, though significant for use of ATMs (automated teller machines) and vending machines, was given lesser weight.

To evaluate feature effectiveness, technical evaluation criteria that were considered included reliability of readings, ease of use, device requirement, applicability to current bills, compatibility with proposed or existing overt security features, ability to cocirculate with current bills, and resistance to simulation. The unit cost of production, capital costs for the BEP and Federal Reserve banks, effects on note durability, feature survivability, availability for immediate or near-term implementation, and experience as proven banknote technology were considered as implementation evaluation criteria. The possibility of incorporation of a feature in the longer term with some additional development or research was also considered.

Further criteria were used for features that required the use of a device. Device criteria included the ability to recognize and denominate banknotes; accuracy, that is, the number of false positives and false negatives; portability; size; maintenance; cost; response time; power use; and longevity. Ability to authenticate was considered to be an important aspect of future development of devices. The output characteristics for devices should consider potential usage by non-English speakers and should take audible (multilingual), tactile, or visual form. Such devices might find application as point-of-sale aids for cash-accepting machines, which would reduce their unit cost.

COMMITTEE FINDINGS

The committee identified three features useful to visually disabled people that can be incorporated in U.S. banknotes without significant further research: banknote size that differs with denomination, large numerals indicating denomination, and banknote color that differs with banknote denomination. The committee received strong support from representatives of organizations of and for visually disabled people for all three of these features. These features are all used in some form in currencies of other countries, and the technology for production is available today.

Because of the status of the ongoing redesign of the U.S. banknotes, the committee is concerned that features not included in the current redesign will not be implemented until a following redesign. The current design sequence will be complete with the issue of the redesigned bill of the smallest denomination in 2001.

Recommended Features Available Now

To ease denomination of U.S. banknotes, the committee recommends the following features (presented in the order in which they are described in the text, with no priority implied):

- *Banknote size as a key to denomination*. Variation of both length and height would allow for more reliable absolute judgment about denomination, while variation of a single dimension would require a secondary cue, such as a size template, to achieve the same level of reliability.
- *Large, high-contrast numerals on a uniform background*. A large, open space will be required in the banknote design to allow for at least a single numeral, in a plain font, that is larger than one-half the current banknote height.
- *Different predominant colors for each of the six denominations printed*. A single color should dominate at least one face of the banknote and should be sufficiently distinguishable from the other colors in the banknote sequence to remain identifiable even in low lighting.
- *Overt features that could lead to the development of effective, low-cost devices for examining banknotes*. Inclusion of a denomination code is recommended to provide for development of devices for those who have difficulty using the recommended features and to add to the ability of visually disabled people to authenticate banknotes.

Findings and Issues Regarding Recommended Features

- All three of these features will serve the majority of the visually disabled—those with low vision. However, of the three features identified, banknote size that differs with denomination is the only one applicable to the needs of blind people.

- Large numerals and color, if applied in a distinct area, may also be used to indicate banknote orientation. No orientation information is given by different-sized banknotes.
- The Treasury Department should evaluate current approaches and conduct studies to determine the sizing needs of each denomination if the six denominations are to be sufficiently distinguishable. This may require, for instance, starting the sequence with a larger $100 banknote.
- The Treasury Department and the Federal Reserve should identify issues regarding the infrastructure of cash-handling machines to determine an appropriate timetable for the introduction of size-denominated banknotes.
- Development of features building on the substantial literature on visual and tactile processes and perception is warranted for near-term feature additions to banknotes. Highly directed, psychophysical/empirical technical work that addresses questions regarding optimum dimensions, optical contrast, location, colors, physical size, etc., for banknote applications should be undertaken.
- Specification of new or enhanced features should not be aimed at minimal levels of recognition performance (i.e., threshold levels) but should strive for sufficient differentiation to permit rapid, relatively effortless performance, with differences between denominations designed to be several times greater than the difference threshold.
- The committee recommends that research be performed to identify combinations of features that enhance denomination and orientation and, perhaps, authentication.
- In reviewing the needs of the 3.7 million U.S. citizens with low vision, the committee observed that many documents issued by government agencies, such as passports, visas, postage stamps, and food stamps, could better serve those with low vision if features similar to those discussed in the report were incorporated in their design. Indeed, in some cases, features not considered sufficiently

robust for application in banknote design might find early application in other government documents.

- The public education campaign accompanying any introduction of new banknote features for visually disabled people would provide a good opportunity for the private sector to consider these types of features for packaging design and related applications.

Recommended Features Requiring Some Additional Research and Development

- The committee urges research on the development of durable tactile features, such as ones printed with "transparent" ink. Transparent-ink tactile marks can be implemented with minimal design changes and so offer flexibility in timing the feature's incorporation.
- The committee recommends research into the implementation issues of holes to denominate banknotes, including the production of durable holes and the psychological questions regarding issuing and using banknotes containing holes.

Research and Development Opportunities

- The committee recommends research to define the threshold and accuracy of reading for the types of low-relief tactile features that are likely to be applicable to banknotes.
- The committee recommends research in the area of enhanced threads, planchettes, or films that would improve devices for examining banknotes.
- The committee recommends that long-term research into advanced features be initiated as possible directions become evident from technology development.
- The committee recommends that analysis regarding the incorporation of advances in microelectronics, nanotechnology,

molecular electronics, materials, photonics, and magnetics in device development be an ongoing effort. Research and development efforts directed toward deriving very sophisticated but inexpensive, reliable, accurate, and inconspicuous devices should be encouraged.

- The BEP should follow the technical work underway by organizations and institutions concerned with the problems of people who are visually disabled and their proposed solutions to those problems, and it should develop a process to assess the applicability of progress in these areas to banknote production.

Implementation Strategies

If the features incorporated in a new design are to be maximally effective, a carefully planned implementation strategy must be developed as the features are evaluated and considered for inclusion. Important aspects of an implementation strategy include the following:

- In selecting features for implementation, the Treasury Department and the Federal Reserve should involve appropriate user groups as early as possible to ensure selection of those features most likely to be used by, and useful to, the target population. The design of any field test should include a cross-section of the target population appropriate to the feature being tested.
- The field test should be broad enough in scope to show not only that the new feature permits recognition under optimal conditions but that rapid, relatively effortless and confidential currency identification are possible across a wide range of everyday circumstances.
- Data gathered from focus groups should be used to help guide the public education campaign that must be a part of the implementation of any new currency feature.
- An appropriate schedule for any introduction of graded sizes of banknotes follows that planned by the BEP for the banknote redesign, beginning with the $100. Since this banknote would be the

largest in the series and represents the smallest production volume, gradual introduction of size-denominated banknotes over the course of six to seven years would allow time for the commercial currency handling industry to prepare for the change.

- In the early stages of distributing sized banknotes, templates would have to be made available to visibly disabled people. The templates might be distributed through banks or appropriate organizations of visually disabled people.

REFERENCES

Benson, V., and M.A. Marano. 1994. Current estimates from the National Health Interview Survey. National Center for Health Statistics, January 1994. Vital and Health Statistics Series 10(189):95.

EBU (European Blind Union). 1994. A report of the European Blind Union Expert Working Group on Currency: Recommendations for the Design of the ECU. Paris, France: EBU.

Genensky, S. 1994. Personal communication to the Committee on Currency Features Usable by the Visually Impaired. March 30, 1994.

NRC (National Research Council). 1993. Counterfeit Deterrent Features for the Next-Generation Currency Design. National Materials Advisory Board, NRC. Washington, D.C.: National Academy Press.

APPENDIX B: SYNOPSIS OF NATIONAL MATERIALS ADVISORY BOARD REPORT 472, COUNTERFEIT DETERRENT FEATURES FOR THE NEXT-GENERATION CURRENCY DESIGN

This study began in 1992 when the Department of Treasury's Bureau of Engraving and Printing requested that the National Research Council, through its National Materials Advisory Board, analyze and recommend overt counterfeit-deterrent features that could be incorporated into the redesign of U.S. banknotes. The major objectives of this study were to:

- analyze and recommend new overt counterfeit-deterrence features that could be incorporated into U.S. currency in the short term, intermediate term, and long term; and
- assess technological directions of future reprographic techniques that could be used for counterfeiting by "casual" and "professional" counterfeiters.

A committee of 12 volunteers with expertise in advanced reprographic technology, chemistry, color, optical science and engineering, paper, physics, security marking, and systems engineering was formed. The Committee on Next-Generation Currency Design met six times between June 1992 and June 1993. Invited presentations by experts from industry and government provided data relevant to the production and inspection of banknotes, advanced reprographic technology,and advanced counterfeit-deterrence features and methods.

This appendix is a summary of the major findings and recommendations of the committee; information regarding counterfeiting threats, feature description and assessment, deterrent strategies, and advances in reprographic technology can be found in the report.

SYNOPSIS

Traditional counterfeiting deterrents, such as unique high-quality paper, fine-line engravings, and high-pressure (intaglio) printing, were adequate in the past to restrict counterfeiting to the dedicated craftsman with access to a printing press; these have kept counterfeiting to a reasonably manageable level in the United States. However, with the advent of advanced reprographic systems, such as color copiers and scanner/computer/printer systems, these methods are no longer sufficient. Widespread availability of these systems, reproduction quality, ease of use, and relative freedom from discovery combine to create an atmosphere for occasional, casual counterfeiting—a crime of opportunity. These systems also provide a convenient base technology for the more professional counterfeiters, so that they need only concentrate on simulating the deterrent features and not on the engraving and printing processes. The counterfeiter's task is made easier by a public in the United States that, for a variety of reasons, does not appear to aggressively examine its banknotes and report counterfeit bills.

Placement of new nonimpact color copier and printer systems in 1995 is expected to exceed 2 million units in the United States, and a similar number is expected for the rest of the world. The number of counterfeit notes produced using nonimpact reprographic technology (i.e., copiers, scanners, and computer printers) is presently small in contrast to that produced by lithographic processes that use specialized equipment. The rate of growth, however, is geometrical. An illustration of how large the problem could become would be to assume that the rate of counterfeiting with nonimpact reprographic equipment doubles every year until year 2000, as it has since 1989. With this assumption, the present-day value of counterfeit currency could grow to almost $2 billion in the year 2000. Such a large amount of counterfeiting would cause severe problems for the economy, as well as impact the ability of law-enforcement agencies to respond. Fortunately, appropriate actions can be taken long before counterfeiting becomes a problem of such proportions.

Over the course of this study, technical information about numerous deterrent features was gathered from vendors, expert witnesses, the Bureau of Engraving and Printing, the Federal Reserve Board, and the Secret Service. This information ranged from conceptual proposals with little or no supporting data to prototypes with extensive test results. A limited amount of data was also available for features already in use on the currency of other countries.

The overall effectiveness of an individual feature was determined by two primary considerations: resistance against technical threat and technical success probability. Resistance against technical threat assumes success in deploying the deterrent and is a measure of the feature's value as a counterfeit deterrent. This category is subdivided into four subcategories: (1) visual and tactile recognizability, (2) inherent resistance to copying, (3) resistance to simulation, and (4) ease of machine readability.

Technical success probability is a measure of the risk of incorporating a feature into a banknote. This category is also subdivided into four subcategories to identify the primary areas of consideration. These are (1) availability and manufacturability, (2) change to recurring production costs, (3) durability, and (4) capital cost of new or modified production tooling.

The two categories, with their eight subcategories, form the cornerstone of the committee's evaluation by helping identify the relative strengths and weaknesses of each feature. The committee did not expect that any single feature would rank first in all categories, and none did. Hence, the committee thought it was important to understand the intent (target) of each deterrent. The committee believed that, in order to provide a multifaceted system of deterrents, consideration should be given to deploying multiple features that complement each other. A well-designed set would address issues of visibility and recognizability under different viewing conditions; require different methods and skills for simulation; and, generally, require too many additional process steps for anyone but the dedicated professional to attempt. Some caution is required, however. The use of too many features could overwhelm the public and thereby reduce the overall effectiveness of the deterrents.

Features that defeat the casual counterfeiter do not necessarily work effectively against professional counterfeiters. Casual, opportunistic counterfeiters do not have the skills, resources, or determination to defeat sophisticated individual deterrents or combinations of them, whereas professional counterfeiters do have these skills and the resources to simulate or duplicate any single deterrent, and probably most combinations, given sufficient time. Certain combinations of features, rather than features acting alone, offer robust potential for defeating the casual counterfeiter and slowing down the professional. In the committee's opinion, the set of deterrent features need not be the same on all denominations of banknotes. For example, more sophisticated features may be used on the $100 banknote than on a $5 (or $1) note.

RECOMMENDATIONS

Although there are many new features that can be used to deter counterfeiters, the Bureau of Engraving and Printing should continue to utilize fine-line engraving, intaglio printing on high-quality pale-tinted paper, and the security thread as methods of deterrence against "classical" printing technologies and present-day reprographics. Future banknote designs should also incorporate additional visible features to serve as deterrents against counterfeiting and as a means for rapid visual authentication. If analysis shows it is cost-effective to do so, some of these overt features could be incorporated into a banknote and their existence not publicly disclosed until they are needed to thwart a new counterfeiting threat.

The BEP should implement a system of complementary features on each banknote that create added complexity for simulation by all levels of counterfeiters. They should not, however, constrain their design by a requirement that the same set of counterfeit-deterrence features be on all denominations of bills.

The BEP should redesign U.S. banknotes to include at least some of these recommended features, making such changes in appearance as are necessary to produce a new series of notes that effectively and efficiently incorporates these advanced counterfeiting deterrents. The recommended features fall into three categories: near term, intermediate term, and long term.

In the near term, the committee recommends incorporation of at least some of the following visible features:

- color-shifting inks for printing;
- moire (alias-generating) line structures, with color added as necessary to enhance the effect;
- security-thread modifications (e.g., with location or width based on the denomination;
- variable-size dot patterns, with color added to enhance the effect; and
- localized watermarks.

For the intermediate term, features requiring inexpensive visual aids for detection at the point of sale are recommended. These include:

- infrared inks for printing;
- optically active coated fibers and particles embedded in the substrate; and
- photoluminescent inks for printing.

Longer-term plans for advanced deterrents should include additional development and understanding of the following features:

- diffraction-based holograms and related devices;
- embedded zero-order diffraction gratings;
- laminated paper substrates with selected features;
- metallic or specular woven security features;
- optical fibers embedded in the substrate; and
- random pattern encryption methods.

For the far term, the Bureau of Engraving and Printing should continually assess fundamental advances in the chemical, applied physical, and biological sciences for developments that are applicable to innovative deterrent features. Assessment of research in psychophysics would also be pertinent, since a better understanding of how people perceive visible features may provide insight into the selection of the "best" features.

Before any new counterfeit-deterrent feature is implemented, it should be evaluated by adversary-analysis experts to determine how readily it can be defeated. This process would be aided by having a means to quickly produce currency with appropriate design changes.

There are other aspects of a counterfeit-deterrent strategy that should be developed along with incorporating new features in banknotes. To begin with, counterfeit-detection education should be emphasized for point-of-sale persons as a priority, and it should be available for the public at large. Potential incentives that would encourage the public to turn in counterfeits should be closely studied to determine which would be effective and not subject to abuse.

Industry should be encouraged to develop effective point-of-sale aids to assist in banknote authentication. Efforts that will lead to a high degree of authentication, particularly for the higher denomination bills, should be continued.

The Department of Treasury should investigate the cost-effectiveness of requiring source identification, such as machine serial numbers, to be embedded in images produced by new copier and printer systems that are capable of producing quality color counterfeit banknotes. If it is determined to be cost-effective, appropriate U.S. legislation requiring source identification should be encouraged. In addition, the Department of Treasury should strongly encourage the use of sensors built into color copier and printer systems that can recognize and inhibit banknote copying. For this approach to be most effective, a unique feature with a high signal-to-noise ratio should be identified, developed, and applied universally to currency, possibly in conjunction with other nations.

To stay ahead of the evolving counterfeiting threats, the Department of Treasury (perhaps led by the Bureau of Engraving and Printing) should establish a multiphased program of identifying and evaluating advances in relevant technologies. Understanding the technological progress in nonimpact printing technologies, and which counterfeiting techniques and methods are being employed, would help the Department of Treasury anticipate advances in the sophistication level of counterfeiters, so that the type and timing of counterfeit deterrents could be planned accordingly. Appropriate mechanisms to accomplish this can take the form of advisory panels, committees, workshops, and briefings.

The Bureau of Engraving and Printing should continue to reevaluate its current materials, process specifications, and tests against actual use requirements, taking into account that different use requirements may apply to different bill denominations. Correlation should be made between the different failure modes of currency experienced in practice and the suite of specification tests performed by the Bureau of Engraving and Printing.

Long-range systematic planning for incorporation of features should be instituted as a regular part of the mission within the Department of Treasury.

Finally, the Department of Treasury should continuously gather data from other nations as to the effectiveness and durability of features such as color-shifting inks and holograms that have been incorporated into their currency.

APPENDIX C: GLOSSARY

Acuity, visual	A measure of the sharpness of an individual's sight compared with that of a "normal" observer. Acuity is measured by finding the smallest letters a person can read at a distance of 20 feet, and expressing the result as the ratio of this distance to the distance at which a "normal" observer can read the same letters.
AMD	Age-related macular degeneration.
ATM	Automated teller machine.
Authenticate	To determine that a banknote is genuine currency.
Banknote	Paper currency.
BEP	Bureau of Engraving and Printing.
Blind	People are said to be blind if with their better eye they have at most light perception. People with this level of visual acuity are sometimes referred to as "functionally blind."
Blind, legally	People are said to be legally blind if the best corrected visual acuity in their better eye does not exceed 20/200, or if the maximum diameter of their visual field does not exceed 20 degrees. This definition is used primarily for official and legal purposes.
Cataract	A form of eye disease that affects vision. Cataracts are opacities within the crystalline lens. The crystalline lens is a structure in the eye between the cornea and the retina. It is an important

Cataract (continued) — optical element in the eye and must remain clear for high quality image formation. Cataracts reduce image quality, often resulting in low-contrast or blurry images. Cataracts are common in old age but are sometimes congenital or arise in conjunction with other eye diseases such as diabetic retinopathy.

Color — The perception in the eye-brain system produced by a nonwhite distribution of electromagnetic energy.

Contrast sensitivity — The ability to perceive small differences in shades of gray. One method for measuring contrast sensitivity is to reduce the contrast of dark letters on a white background until they can no longer be recognized. The lowest contrast at which the letters can be recognized is the threshold level, and the reciprocal of this is the contrast sensitivity.

Covert features — Features that are hidden in the banknote and are not intended to be made public. Used by the Federal Reserve for currency authentication and by law enforcement for forensic purposes.

Currency — Paper money in circulation.

Delaminate — To separate into constituent layers.

Denominate — To determine the value of a banknote.

Disability, visual — Blindness or low vision.

Embedded features — Features that are added during the paper-making process or inserted between laminated layers. They include threads, planchettes, fibers, microtaggants, microcapsules, and so on.

Enhanced fibers — Fibers that respond to ultraviolet, infrared, or other excitations to give identifiable reactions and are added to paper as a security feature.

Fibers — Dyed fibers embedded in the paper as a security feature. See also "Enhanced fibers."

Field, visual — The range of visual directions, centered on the line of sight, over which a standardized test target can be detected.

Fluorescence	The emission of light or other electromagnetic radiation of longer wavelengths by a substance as a result of the absorption of some other radiation of shorter wavelengths, provided the emission continues only as long as the stimulus producing it is maintained. In other words, fluorescence is the luminescence that persists for less than about 10^{-8} s after excitation.
Glare sensitivity	An adverse effect of bright lighting on vision. For example, oncoming headlights at night may adversely affect visibility of the road ahead in someone with glare sensitivity. Early cataracts may result in glare sensitivity.
Glaucoma	Glaucoma is a disease that occurs when the intra-ocular pressure becomes excessively high (due to inadequate drainage of aqueous humor from the anterior chamber of the eye). The excessive pressure can ultimately damage retinal cells, first resulting in loss of peripheral vision and later progressing (if untreated) to encompass the entire visual field.
Intaglio printing	A printing process where characters are formed as depressed areas on the printing plates. These are filled with ink, which is transferred to paper under pressure.
Issuing authority	An entity entitled to officially distribute banknotes.
Laminate	A sheet of material made of one or more bonded layers.
LED	Light-emitting diode.
Letterpress printing	Printing in which characters are formed by raised surfaces on the printing plates; a roller applies ink to these raised surfaces, and the plate is pressed against the paper to transfer the ink.
Light perception	People are said to have, at most, light perception if, with their better eye, they are able to detect the presence of light but are not able to determine the direction from which the light is coming.
Low vision	Best-corrected acuity less than 20/60 in the better eye. Sometimes defined as the inability to read regular newsprint with optimal reading glasses at normal reading distance.
Luminescence	See "Fluorescence" and "Phosphorescence."

Maculopathy	Disease associated with the central (macular) portion of the retina. Maculopathies usually have an adverse effect on high-acuity central vision. Age-related maculopathy is the most common form of low vision and afflicts many older people.
Microcapsules	Small particles, not visible to the eye that are added to substrate and that respond to ultraviolet, infrared, or other excitations to give identifiable reactions.
Overt feature	A feature that is made public and is visible or apparent without requiring special instruments. May require some instruction on how to observe it.
Paper	The substrate used in printing currency, usually based on cotton and linen fibers rather than on cellulose, as in ordinary paper.
Paper furnish	The fiber-water slurry from which the paper is made.
Peripheral field loss	Loss of vision outside of the central region of the visual field. In the extreme, it results in "tunnel vision," in which only a very narrow central region of vision remains.
Phosphorescence	The emission of light or other electromagnetic radiation that is delayed by more than 10^{-8} s following excitation.
Planchettes	Colored or reflective pieces of paper or plastic a few millimeters in diameter that are added during paper manufacture.
Recognize	To identify a piece of paper as a banknote, rather than as a similar sized piece of paper such as a store receipt.
Reprographic	Facsimile reproduction of graphic matter, for example, by photocopying or printing from a computer.
Retinopathy	A noninflammatory retinal disease.
Saturation, color	The degree of purity or chroma.
Security thread	The thread present inside the paper used in currency printing. It may carry the domination of the bill or may be fully metallized.
Substrate	The medium on which currency is printed. May be paper, plastic, or a laminated combination.

Smart Money	A form of currency that contains an encryption or information that can uniquely identify and verify the value of the currency.
Substrate	The medium on which banknotes are printed. May be paper, plastic, or a laminated combination.
Target	A form that an individual wishes to distinguish from its background. Specifically, the numerals on a banknote indicating the denomination.
Target population	A group that will be able to use a particular feature in banknotes.
Thread	See "Security thread."
Usher Syndrome	An inherited disorder characterized by moderate to profound hearing impairment, which is present at birth or shortly thereafter, and by progressive vision loss due to retinitis pigmentosa, a degeneration of the retina.
Visually impaired	A person with any form of visual disability that interferes with daily activities, including people who are blind or have low vision or people with peripheral field deficits, glare sensitivity, or losses in contrast sensitivity.
Watermark	A localized modification of the structure and opacity of a sheet of paper so that the pattern or design can be seen when the sheet is held to the light.

APPENDIX D: FEATURES IN USE WORLDWIDE

There are currently over 180 countries in the world that issue their own banknotes. Of these, around 50 countries print the banknotes internally; the remainder have their banknotes printed by commercial currency security printers under contract. Some countries have specifically addressed the problem of visually disabled people and have striven to add appropriate features. Other countries have coincidentally included effective features in the course of producing an attractive banknote design, although the prime aim was assisting the normally sighted public to handle denominations easily.

BREAKDOWN OF FEATURE TYPES

The existing range of feature types is characterized below. An enlargement of their use in practice is given in the following section.

1. variable-size banknotes;
2. large numerals on banknotes;
3. variable-color banknotes;
4. special shaped patterns;
5. specific engraved visible markings;
6. specific engraved invisible markings;
7. watermark features; and
8. machine-identifiable features.

DESCRIPTION OF FEATURE TYPES

Variable-Size Banknotes

Of the 171 issuing authorities identified by the committee, more than 100 issue banknotes that vary in size for the different denominations. Size variation currently occurs in two forms:

(1) the long edge varies while the short edge remains constant (e.g., in Iceland) or (2) both edges vary (e.g., in England).

Size variation was originally introduced to allow the normally sighted public an easy way to differentiate among denominations. This was particularly useful when the basic design style was common among different denominations. Wallets were produced with different size pockets to enable the banknotes to be easily separated.

Subsequently, it has been found that this is a useful aid to visually disabled people, including the blind population. Simple size gauges have been made that enable the note to be examined by touch against a fixed reference point so that denomination can be determined. Recently there has been a worldwide trend toward reducing the size of banknotes for cost-related reasons. This has been mainly caused by rising inflation leading to an increased need for ever higher denomination banknotes and, hence, extra-large sizes. Where size variation within a denominational structure exists, it has been retained for any new family of notes.

Large Numerals on Banknotes

Banknote designers have often considered it important to ensure that the denomination in numerals, rather than in text, is displayed in a prominent position. The size of the numerals has depended on the overall design style and the number of repetitions of the denomination on each face of the note. With fewer repetitions, it has been possible to incorporate larger numerals.

The presence of large numerals helps both the normally sighted and the visually disabled public and is an approach that has been taken with increasing frequency in recent years.

The current Dutch series of banknotes has been designed with extremely large central values on both faces. The number value is a predominant part of the design. A more common approach is the use of a single large numeral value, as displayed on the current Czech Republic currency. More and more modern designs are being produced with this type of approach. Of the 171 issuing authorities tabulated in Table D-1 (at the end of this appendix), 24 can be said to have adopted a specific scheme including large numerals in their banknote design.

Variable-Color Banknotes

The currency of the United States is exclusive in the world for its use of common colors front and back for all denominations of banknotes. Even where countries use same-size banknotes for each denomination, they use color as a means of distinguishing the individual value. Of the 171 issuing authorities tabulated below, 167 use a clearly differentiated color scheme for all denominations and an additional two use color for some denominations.

Although people have various degrees of color vision, distinctive color differences among denominations, using appropriately chosen colors, can form a major separation technique for all except blind people. The amount of color difference depends on the individual choice of the country.

Special Shaped Patterns

Besides printing large denominational values to assist certain sections of the visually disabled public, a more recent approach has been to print a distinctively shaped image on each note that changes with the value. The current series from the Bank of England has a solid circle to represent £5, a diamond for £10, a square for £20, and a triangle for £50. The printings are made in strong colors with a clear edge to the shape to aid recognition by the visually disabled population.

Specific Engraved Visible Marks

The use of intaglio printing on currency has long been regarded as a way of providing a tactile feature for blind people. This assumption is based on the fact that blind people use touch to identify the raised characteristics of braille. Since intaglio itself is a three-dimensional printing process, specific identifiers can be included to separate each denomination. The marks have taken the form of small geometric shapes that form different groupings and locations for each denomination. In practice there is a large difference between the relief of an average braille dot above the paper surface (approximately 400 μm) and that of the typical intaglio marks (approximately 40–50 μm). During the course of a banknote's circulated life, as the note becomes worn, the level of the mark's profile becomes reduced. Examples of tactile marks can be seen on the currencies of Germany, the Netherlands, and Malaysia. The survey (Table D-1) indicated that around 16 countries have adopted this approach for each denomination, and a further 7 have a tactile feature on some denominations.

Current thinking in the banknote manufacturing community is that the marks are an attempt to provide a feature useful to visually impaired people, but in practice they are only evident to the normally sighted. Currency design is moving toward the inclusion of large numerals or special shaped patterns.

Specific Engraved Invisible Marks

A recent development in features for visually disabled people can be seen in the Dutch approach to the new 100 Guilder banknote. A large part of the front surface of the note is covered with intaglio printed transparent ink in the form of randomly located dots. This has the merit of enabling a large area of the note to be used for tactile effects without affecting the visual security image.

On the current series, the dots have been included to provide a tactile clue for the presence of genuine currency versus a flat counterfeit. Modification of the area layout could allow for a specific pattern to be included for each denomination. The dots are 1.0 mm in diameter and have a height above the background of 70 μm.

Watermark Images

The Japanese have introduced a set of special geometric watermark shapes in the corner of the note to give assistance in denomination. The watermark has a sharp visual profile that gives a clear image by transmission. The nature and location of the image changes with denomination.

Measurements taken from banknotes have shown that the lighter areas are 50 μm below the average height of the paper. Again this can be compared with the value of 400 μm for braille characters.

Machine-Identifiable Features

The Bank of Canada has a design similar to that of the United States in that it issues common-size dollar bills. When the current series of notes was being developed, particular attention was paid to the problem of the visually disabled population. In addition to using some large numerals and lettering, the bank decided to develop a small hand-held device to ensure a note could be positively identified.

The notes have been designed with specific, large colored patches in the intaglio pattern changing in location on each denomination. A detector was developed that is capable of assessing the presence or absence of the intaglio ink in specific places. By using a simple coding arrangement, it is possible to positively identify the denomination of each note. An audible message is given from the device for the benefit of blind people. Although the unit can discriminate among denominations in genuine currency, it is not to be regarded as an authentication device, as it can be confused by simple black patches drawn on genuine or counterfeit banknotes.

SUMMARY OF FEATURES ON WORLDWIDE CURRENCIES

The following table shows the major features contained in 171 different styles of banknotes around the world. The table is not exhaustive, as some countries issue more than one style of note (e.g., Scotland), and the varying political state of the world leads to formation of new countries where currency details are limited (e.g., the former Yugoslavia). The term "issuing authority" indicates that the entity described has permission to design and print currency but may not be a sovereign country. For example, the Isle of Man, Guernsey, Northern Ireland, England, and Scotland each issue banknotes exchangeable throughout the United Kingdom. All are considered issuing authorities, but not all are independent countries.

Some of the currencies described in Table D-1 are no longer issued but are included as examples of currency in circulation around the world. The number of denominations currently issued is included where known. When countries issue banknotes with new designs, the new notes generally cocirculate with the old-design notes, which can result in as many as 20 different banknotes being legal tender at any one time.

CONCLUDING OBSERVATIONS

It can be seen that a number of different approaches have been used to provide banknotes more suitable to the visually disabled population. However, no single approach has emerged as the standard for all notes worldwide. This has to do with issues of tradition as well as issues of viability.

REFERENCES

Haslop, J.M. 1994. Personal communication to the Committee on Currency Features Usable by the Visually Impaired. August 1994.

Table D-1 Summary of Currency Features for Visually Disabled People Used in Currency from 171 Issuing Authorities Around the World

Issuing Authority	Number of Denominations	Denomination Differentiation Method (Y = yes; N = no; S = some denominations)			
		Color	Size	Tactile Recognition Symbol	Large Numeral
Afghanistan	6	Y	S	N	S
Albania	4	Y	Y	N	N
Algeria	4	Y	S	N	N
Angola	6	Y	Y	N	N
Argentina	7	Y	N	Y	Y
Armenia	6	Y	S	Y	N
Aruba	5	Y	N	Y	Y
Australia	5	Y	Y	N	S
Austria	6	Y	Y	Y	N
Bahamas	7	Y	N	N	Y
Bahrain	5	Y	S	N	N
Bangladesh	7	Y	Y	N	N
Barbados	6	Y	N	N	N
Belgium	6	Y	Y	Y	Y
Belize	6	Y	N	N	N
Bermuda	6	Y	N	N	N
Bolivia	5	Y	N	N	S
Botswana	5	Y	Y	N	S
Brazil	6	Y	N	N	S
Brunei	7	Y	Y	N	N
Bulgaria	5	Y	Y	Y	Y
Burundi	5	Y	Y	N	S
Cambodia	7	Y	Y	N	N
Cameroon	5	Y	Y	N	N
Canada	7	Y	N	N	Y

Table D-1 Summary of Currency Features for Visually Disabled People Used in Currency from 171 Issuing Authorities Around the World (continued)

Issuing Authority	Number of Denominations	Denomination Differentiation Method (Y = yes; N = no; S = some denominations)			
		Color	Size	Tactile Recognition Symbol	Large Numeral
Cape Verde	5	Y	Y	N	N
Cayman Islands	4	Y	N	N	N
Central African Republic	5	Y	S	N	N
Chad	5	Y	Y	N	N
Chile	4	Y	N	N	N
China	6	Y	S	Y	N
Colombia	7	Y	N	S	N
Comoros	3	Y	Y	N	N
Congo	5	Y	Y	N	N
Cook Islands	4	Y	N	N	N
Costa Rica	5	Y	N	N	N
Croatia	11	Y	S	Y	N
Cuba	7	Y	N	N	N
Cyprus	5	Y	Y	S	N
Czech Republic	6	Y	Y	Y	N
Denmark	5	Y	S	N	N
Djibouti	5	Y	Y	N	N
Dominican Republic	8	Y	N	N	N
Eastern Caribbean Territories	5	Y	N	N	N
Ecuador	9	Y	N	N	N
Egypt	6	Y	S	N	N
El Salvador	7	S	Y	N	N
England	4	Y	Y	Y	N
Equatorial Guinea	4	Y	Y	N	N
Estonia	7	Y	N	N	S

Table D-1 Summary of Currency Features for Visually Disabled People Used in Currency from 171 Issuing Authorities Around the World (continued)

Issuing Authority	Number of Denominations	Denomination Differentiation Method (Y = yes; N = no; S = some denominations)			
		Color	Size	Tactile Recognition Symbol	Large Numeral
Ethiopia	5	Y	Y	N	N
Falkland Islands	4	Y	N	N	N
Faroe Islands	7	Y	Y	N	N
Fiji	5	Y	Y	N	N
Finland	6	Y	N	N	N
France	5	Y	Y	N	S
French Territories in the Pacific	4	Y	Y	N	N
Gabon	5	Y	Y	N	N
Gambia	5	Y	Y	N	N
Germany	8	Y	Y	S	S
Ghana	6	Y	S	N	N
Gibraltar	5	Y	Y	N	N
Greece	5	Y	Y	N	N
Guatemala	7	Y	N	N	N
Guernsey	4	Y	Y	N	N
Guinea	6	Y	Y	N	N
Guinea-Bissau	6	Y	Y	N	N
Guyana	5	Y	N	N	N
Haiti	9	Y	S	N	N
Honduras	6	Y	Y	N	N
Hong Kong	5	Y	Y	N	N
Hungary	5	Y	N	N	N
Iceland	6	Y	Y	N	N
India	7	Y	S	N	N
Indonesia	7	Y	Y	N	N

Table D-1 Summary of Currency Features for Visually Disabled People Used in Currency from 171 Issuing Authorities Around the World (continued)

Issuing Authority	Number of Denominations	Denomination Differentiation Method (Y = yes; N = no; S = some denominations)			
		Color	Size	Tactile Recognition Symbol	Large Numeral
Iran	7	Y	Y	N	N
Iraq	6	Y	Y	N	N
Ireland	4	Y	Y	N	N
Israel	7	Y	N	Y	N
Italy	6	Y	Y	N	N
Jamaica	7	Y	S	N	N
Japan	6	Y	Y	N	N
Jersey	5	Y	Y	N	N
Jordan	5	Y	Y	N	N
Kazakstan	8	Y	S	N	N
Kenya	6	Y	Y	N	N
Korea (South)	4	Y	Y	N	N
Kuwait	5	Y	Y	N	N
Laos	5	Y	Y	N	N
Lebanon	9	Y	Y	N	N
Lesotho	5	Y	Y	N	N
Libya	5	Y	Y	N	N
Lithuania	6	Y	N	N	N
Luxembourg	3	Y	Y	N	N
Macao	6	Y	Y	N	N
Madagascar	6	Y	S	N	N
Malawi	6	Y	Y	N	N
Malaysia	8	Y	Y	S	N
Maldives	7	Y	N	N	N
Mali	5	Y	Y	N	N

Table D-1 Summary of Currency Features for Visually Disabled People Used in Currency from 171 Issuing Authorities Around the World (continued)

Issuing Authority	Number of Denominations	Denomination Differentiation Method (Y = yes; N = no; S = some denominations)			
		Color	Size	Tactile Recognition Symbol	Large Numeral
Malta	4	Y	Y	N	N
Man (Isle of)	4	Y	Y	N	N
Mauritania	4	S	Y	N	N
Mauritius	8	Y	Y	N	N
Mexico	8	Y	N	N	N
Mongolia	8	Y	Y	N	N
Morocco	4	Y	Y	S	N
Mozambique	6	Y	S	N	N
Myanmar	7	Y	Y	N	N
Macedonia	5	Y	N	N	N
Namibia	3	Y	Y	Y	N
Nepal	8	Y	Y	N	N
Netherlands	7	Y	Y	S	S
Netherlands Antilles	6	Y	N	Y	N
New Zealand	5	Y	Y	N	N
Nicaragua	9	Y	N	N	N
Nigeria	5	Y	N	N	N
Northern Ireland	5	Y	Y	N	N
Norway	4	Y	Y	N	N
Oman	9	Y	Y	N	N
Pakistan	7	Y	Y	N	N
Papua New Guinea	4	Y	S	N	N
Paraguay	7	Y	S	N	N
Peru	6	Y	S	S	N
Philippines	7	Y	N	N	N

Table D-1 Summary of Currency Features for Visually Disabled People Used in Currency from 171 Issuing Authorities Around the World (continued)

Issuing Authority	Number of Denominations	Denomination Differentiation Method (Y = yes; N = no; S = some denominations)			
		Color	Size	Tactile Recognition Symbol	Large Numeral
Poland	11	Y	N	N	S
Portugal	5	Y	Y	N	N
Qatar	6	Y	Y	N	N
Romania	7	Y	Y	N	N
Russia	7	Y	S	N	S
Rwanda	4	Y	Y	N	N
Saint Helena	4	Y	Y	N	N
Sao Tome and Principe	4	Y	Y	N	N
Saudi Arabia	6	Y	Y	N	N
Scotland	5	Y	S	N	N
Seychelles	4	Y	N	N	N
Sierra Leone	8	Y	N	N	N
Singapore	7	Y	Y	N	N
Slovenia	8	Y	Y	N	N
Solomon Islands	5	Y	Y	N	N
Somalia	5	Y	S	N	N
South Africa	3	Y	Y	Y	S
Spain	4	Y	Y	N	N
Sri Lanka	7	Y	Y	N	N
Sudan	7	Y	N	N	S
Surinam	6	Y	N	N	S
Swaziland	5	N	Y	N	N
Sweden	6	Y	Y	N	N
Switzerland	6	Y	Y	Y	Y
Syria	7	Y	Y	N	N

Table D-1 Summary of Currency Features for Visually Disabled People Used in Currency from 171 Issuing Authorities Around the World (continued)

Issuing Authority	Number of Denominations	Denomination Differentiation Method (Y = yes; N = no; S = some denominations)			
		Color	Size	Tactile Recognition Symbol	Large Numeral
Taiwan	6	Y	S	N	N
Tanzania	6	Y	Y	N	N
Thailand	7	Y	Y	N	N
Tonga	6	Y	N	N	N
Trinidad and Tobago	5	Y	N	N	N
Tunisia	3	Y	Y	N	N
Turkey	6	Y	Y	N	N
Uganda	8	Y	S	N	N
United Arab Emirates	6	Y	Y	N	N
United States of America	6	N	N	N	N
Uruguay	7	Y	N	Y	N
Vanuatu	4	Y	Y	N	N
Venezuela	6	Y	N	N	N
Vietnam	11	Y	Y	N	N
West African Monetary Union	5	Y	Y	N	N
Western Samoa	4	Y	Y	N	N
Yemen	6	Y	Y	N	N
Yugoslavia	8	Y	Y	N	N
Zaire	8	Y	Y	N	N
Zambia	5	Y	Y	N	N
Zimbabwe	4	Y	Y	N	N

APPENDIX E: FEATURES NOT SUBJECT TO FULL EVALUATION

During the course of its deliberations, the committee identified a number of potential ideas that did not warrant full evaluation. As an aid to any future discussions of this topic, these ideas have been identified in tabular form below, together with the reason why they were not taken further.

Table E-1 Features Not Subjected to a Full Evaluation

Feature	Rationale
Variable edge texture as in coins	The thickness of a banknote does not provide sufficient area for discrimination, and there is a limited technical probability of success.
Holes of different shapes	Although the principle of holes is covered in detail, the concept of using differently shaped holes was rejected on grounds that, with wear, any shaped hole will become rounded and will lose its distinction.
Paper snap or handle	Although currency paper has a distinctive crackle, it was not considered feasible to provide a range of sound options.
Different basis weight	The committee considered that the range of basis weight values required to provide an acceptable discrimination to the untrained public over six values would range from tissue paper to board.

Table E-1 Features Not Subjected to a Full Evaluation (continued)

Feature	Rationale
Use of superabsorbents	The idea of introducing superabsorbent material that could expand on water contact and produce localized tactile marks was considered potentially useful. However, the idea was rejected, as it was not considered feasible to get 100 percent reversibility.
Laminated structures with debonded areas	Although considered as an approach to tactile effect, no technology was identified that was capable of introducing this approach.
Variable stiffness	The idea of creating different denominations with different stiffness was put forward. However, it is well known that current banknotes vary in stiffness during the normal circulation due to wear. It was therefore considered that this feature would be very difficult to develop.
Windowed thread as used on English currency, with number of windows indicating denomination	This feature would not be suitable for blind people. It would also require large-sized windows to assist visually impaired people. This would not be possible to achieve on the normal height of notes and still give adequate durability.
Laminated sheet with localized punchings on end side with rough center	From evidence of tactile perception, this was considered unrealistic for the untrained person to identify, especially where considerations of wear were taken into account.
Acoustic effect from edge of bill	The possibility of each denomination causing a different sound when dragged over a surface or blown on the edges was considered. However, the technology was considered impractical at the current time.

Table E-1 Features Not Subjected to a Full Evaluation (continued)

Feature	Rationale
Papers with different porosity that would be identified by blowing air through them	Existing banknotes vary in porosity during the course of their lifetime. The possibility of controlling this parameter within boundaries that were even machine detectable was considered unrealistic.
Piezoelectric effects	Although natural fibers are know to encompass piezoelectric characteristics, it was considered that the variations required when, for example, bending the note, were beyond current identification technology.
Olfactory detection	The possibility of impregnating notes with a microencapsulated odor was considered impractical at present. Problems of durability and cross odor contamination eliminated this approach.
Shape (triangular, circular, etc.)	The idea of having variously shaped currency was considered impractical from a manufacturing and handling standpoint.
Patches applied after banknote manufacture, indicating denomination by location or texture	The idea of adding features after banknote manufacture was considered impractical for two reasons. First a large, localized area 100 μm or more above the banknote "background" would create problems (including durability of banknotes, adherence of the patch, and jamming of machines) with automated cash-handling machines and of uneven stacking. Second, there is concern about the security implications of having to match a separate patch with a banknote after printing processes are completed.
Thin silicon chip	This technology is not considered advanced enough for incorporation now.

APPENDIX F: DESCRIPTION OF THE NEW DESIGN CONCEPT

On July 13, 1994, the Secretary of the Treasury announced a new design concept for the $100 banknote, due for production by 1996. The lower denomination banknotes will also be redesigned. These will be introduced at the rate of approximately one new denomination design per year. Since the design for the $100 notes was announced prior to completion of this study, it does not incorporate the recommendations included in this report. Several new features in the new design are of interest to the current study, so a brief description of the new design is included in this report.

In addition to traditional numerals, titles, and engraved borders similar to the current design, the new design will have a larger, off-center portrait and a portrait watermark (see Figure F-1). In addition, several other features have been chosen for inclusion in the design. All of these features will require some development and feasibility analysis, so the final design chosen after all the development work may not contain all the features proposed in the original design. These features are as follows:

- *Distinctive, machine-detectable fibers*. Special fibers with specific properties are often added to security papers for forensic purposes. Modern security fibers can be designed to incorporate many types of machine-detectable characteristics.
- *Iridescent planchettes*. Traditional planchettes are colored pieces of tissue paper a few millimeters in diameter incorporated directly into the paper, either in rows or randomly distributed. In newer planchettes, such features as microprinting and iridescence are used to enhance the security.
- *Security thread*: A security thread is a thin thread or ribbon running through a banknote substrate. It is a versatile feature, and there are many types currently available, including microprinted, metallic, magnetic, windowed, and imbedded. The thread currently in use in U.S. currency is an embedded, microprinted thread that can only be seen when held to light. This characteristic makes it impossible to copy with a color copier, which uses reflected light to generate an image.
- *Watermark*. A watermark is an image formed by purposely creating localized variations in the paper density during the papermaking process. The image is visible as darker and lighter areas when held against a light source. Like the embedded thread, it does not copy on color copiers.

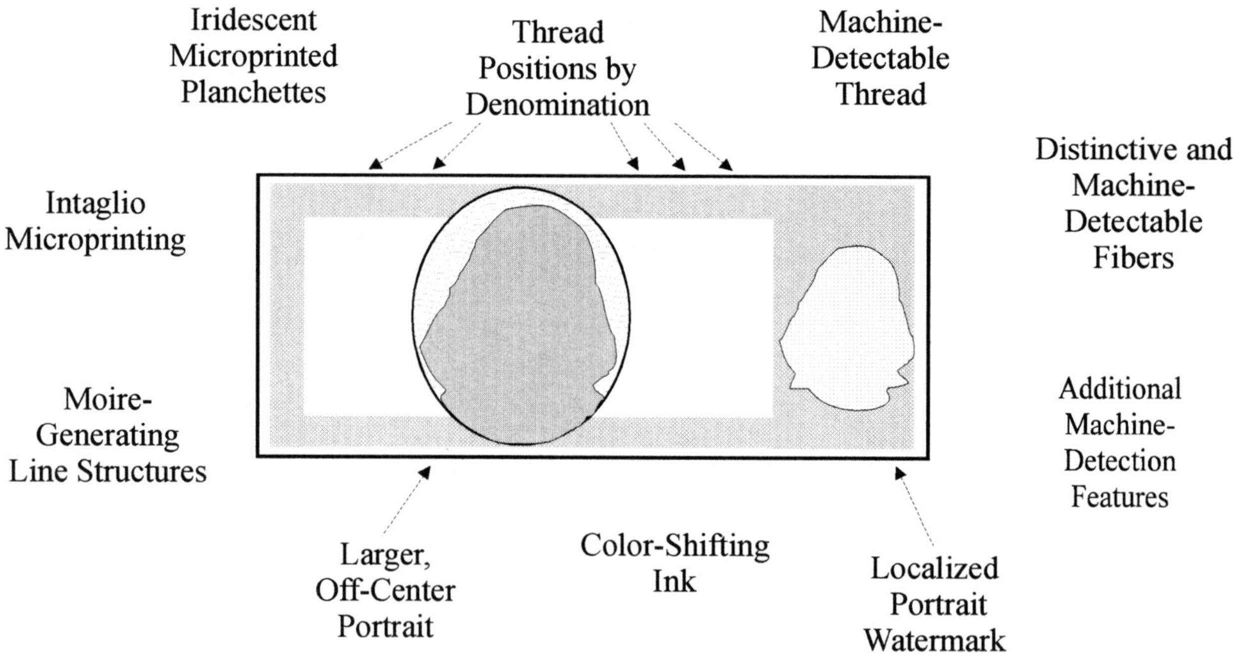

Shaded portions indicate areas for numerals, titles and traditional engraved borders.

Figure F-1 Design concept for the new $100 bill, as introduced by the Department of the Treasury.

- *Color-shifting inks.* These inks change color when viewed from different angles. For instance, an ink that appears gold when viewed directly may change to green when viewed obliquely.
- *Moiré-generating line structures.* These types of line structures appear normal to the human eye but cannot be properly resolved by scanning equipment. This results in the creation of spurious images, or moiré patterns, in the digital output, producing a copy that is noticeably distinguishable from the original.

APPENDIX G: BIOGRAPHIES OF COMMITTEE MEMBERS

NORBERT S. BAER received his M.S. from the University of Wisconsin and his Ph.D. from New York University in physical chemistry. His research interests include the application of physicochemical methods to the examination and preservation of artistic and historical works. In 1980 he chaired the National Materials Advisory Board Committee on Conservation of Historic Stone Buildings and Monuments and since 1980 has chaired the National Archives Advisory Committee on Preservation. He served on the National Materials Advisory Board from 1986 to 1993. From 1983 to 1984 Dr. Baer was a John Simon Guggenheim Memorial Foundation Fellow. From 1985 to 1986 he served as Technical Advisor to the National Materials Advisory Board's Committee on Preservation of Historical Records. He is currently Hagop Kevorkian Professor of Conservation at New York University. Dr. Baer was a member of the Committee on Next-Generation Currency Design.

GARY A. BAUM received his B.S. from the University of Wisconsin and his M.S. and Ph.D. from Oklahoma State University. His industrial research experience began in 1963 when he joined the Douglas Aircraft Company as a research engineer. He joined Dow Chemical Company and then moved to the Institute of Paper Chemistry, where he became professor of physics and director of the Paper Materials Division. Dr. Baum then joined James River Corporation and moved into the position of Director of Corporate Research and Development. He is a fellow of the Technical Association of the Pulp and Paper Industry and has served on their board of directors. He is currently head of the Department of Wood and Paper Science, North Carolina State University, Raleigh.

JOHN A. BRABYN received his B.E. with First Class Honors in Electrical Engineering from the University of Canterbury, Christchurch, New Zealand. He pursued studies of electronic mobility aids for the blind, gaining a Ph.D. degree in electrical engineering in 1978. His interest in technology for the blind was continued at the Smith-Kettlewell Eye Research Institute starting in 1978, where he developed the first phased-array scanning air sonar and designed and built an interface between that device and a tactile display for blind pedestrians. Subsequently, he became co-director of the Smith-Kettlewell Rehabilitation Engineering Research Center for the Blindness and Low Vision, where he has participated in and coordinated a large number of projects in technology for the blind, including devices for orientation and mobility, braille literacy, vocational applications, low vision, and communication for individuals who are both deaf and blind. Dr. Brabyn currently holds the positions of senior scientist at the Kettlewell-Eye Research Institute and co-director of the Rehabilitation Engineering Research Center. He has served on numerous national review bodies and advisory boards, including as chair of the National Eye Institute Special Study Section for Small Business Innovative Research from 1986 to 1992. He is the author of many scientific journal articles and conference presentations on technology for the blind and visually impaired.

JOSEPH GAYNOR received his B.Ch.E. from Polytechnic Institute Brooklyn (now Polytechnic University) and a Ph.D. from Case Institute of Technology (now Case-Western Reserve University). His technical interests and expertise include areas such as imaging materials and processes, nonimpact printing technologies, optical memory materials and processes, chemical processes, photochemistry (especially applications), and polymeric films and coatings. He was a member of two former National Materials Advisory Board committees (1984–1987, 1992–1993) concerned with U.S. currency. He is president of Innovative Technologies Associates in Ventura, California.

JOHN M. HASLOP received his M.Tech. in applied chemistry from Brunel University, England. He joined Metal Box Company in 1961 and worked on various aspects of commercial packaging print application. Since 1965 he has been employed by Thomas De La Rue and Company Limited. His research interests are in ink formulation and product development for all types of security documents and printing processes. He is a member of the Royal Chemical Society, the Institute of Printing, and the Forensic Science Society. At various times, he has been responsible for factory liaison, technical marketing of the banknote product, and—for fourteen years—management of the research and development group. Mr. Haslop currently occupies the position of divisional technical manager, Thomas De La Rue and Company, Basingstoke, Hampshire, England.

GORDON E. LEGGE received his S.B. in physics from the Massachusetts Institute of Technology in 1971, his M.A. in astronomy from Harvard University in 1972, and his Ph.D. in experimental psychology in 1976. His research interests are in visual perception, with specialty areas of everyday tasks and low vision. Dr. Legge is also interested in topics in cognitive science, including reading and object recognition. He has served on numerous boards and done consulting work in these areas for various academic and industrial organizations. He is a member of the American Association for the Advancement of Science and a member of the Association for Research in Vision and Opththalmology. Dr. Legge is the winner of the 1994 Pisart Lighthouse Vision Award. He is presently director of the Minnesota Laboratory for Low-Vision Research and a professor in the Department of Psychology, University of Minnesota.

ROBERT R. SHANNON received his B.S. and M.A. from the University of Rochester. He is an expert in applied optics and is well known for his practical approach to problems. He has both academic and industrial experience. For the past twenty-five years he has been a professor at the University of Arizona and is a past director of the Optical Sciences

Center. He is a member of the National Academy of Engineering and is currently Professor Emeritus at the University of Arizona. He was a member of two former National Materials Advisory Board committees (1984–1987, 1992–1993) concerned with U.S. currency.

GLENN T. SINCERBOX received his B.S. in physics from Rensselaer Polytechnic Institute in 1959 and his M.S. in physics from the University of Illinois in 1960. He continued graduate studies at the University of Illinois until 1962, when he joined IBM. He has been a member of the research staff at IBM's Almaden Research Center since 1972, where he has held several technical and managerial positions. He is currently program manager of holographic storage systems and technology. His primary research contributions have been in the areas of holography, novel recording processes, and optical devices, with emphasis on their application to information storage, display, scanning, printing, and inspection. Mr. Sincerbox has published and presented over 60 papers and 3 book chapters, and he holds 39 patents and over 65 patent publications. He is the recipient of 15 IBM invention achievement awards and an IBM Outstanding Innovation Award. He is a fellow of the Optical Society of America and has served on numerous society and conference committees. Mr. Sincerbox was chair of the 1992–1993 National Materials Advisory Board study on Counterfeit Deterrent Features for the Next-Generation Currency Design and was also a member of the 1985–1987 National Materials Advisory Board studies on currency and counterfeiting.